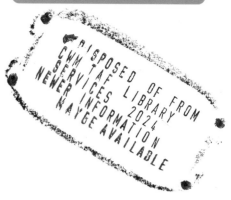
on or before

INTRODUCTION TO
MINIMAL ACCESS SURGERY

INTRODUCTION TO MINIMAL ACCESS SURGERY

Edited by

Timothy H Brown MD, FRCS

Consultant general surgeon, Morriston Hospital NHS Trust, Swansea

and

M H Irving FRCS

Professor of general surgery, Hope Hospital, Salford

First published in 1995
by the BMJ Publishing Group, BMA House, Tavistock Square,
London WC1H 9JR

British Library Cataloguing in Publication Data

A catalogue record for this book is available
from the British Library

ISBN 0-7279-0885-5

Typeset by Latimer Trend & Company Ltd., Plymouth
Printed and bound by Craft Print, Singapore

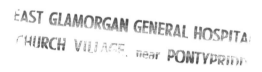

Contents

CONTENTS

Contributors

John Bancewicz, consultant surgeon, Hope Hospital, Salford, Manchester

Mark S Cade, registrar in urology, Leeds General Infirmary

Andrew D Clarke, surgical registrar, Manchester rotation, Manchester

G Griffiths, senior registrar in surgery, Manchester Royal Infirmary

J Hill, consultant surgeon, Manchester Royal Infirmary

T L Hooper, senior lecturer and consultant cardiothoracic surgeon, Wythenshawe Hospital, Manchester

Andrew C Howard, orthopaedic senior registrar, Northern General Hospital, Sheffield

N R Hulton, consultant surgeon, Royal Oldham Hospital, Oldham, Lancashire

Mark T Jones, consultant cardiothoracic surgeon, Wythenshawe Hospital, Manchester

Adrian D Joyce, consultant urologist, Leeds General Infirmary

D D Kerrigan, consultant surgeon, Aintree Centre for GI Oncology, Aintree Hospital NHS Trust, Liverpool

I MacLennan, consultant surgeon, Manchester Royal Infirmary

M M Mughal, consultant surgeon, Chorley and District Hospital, Chorley, Lancashire

R C Pearson, consultant surgeon, Manchester Royal Infirmary

Timothy J Rockley, consultant ENT surgeon, Burton Hospitals NHS Trust,
    Burton-on-Trent, Staffordshire

Nigel A Scott, consultant surgeon, Hope Hospital, Salford, Manchester

A R B Smith, consultant gynaecologist, St Mary's Hospital for Women and Children, Whitworth Park, Manchester

Foreword

Ever since the dawn of civilisation, advances in technology and advances in surgery have been inseparably linked. A glance at ancient text books of surgery reveals examples of the ingenuity of surgeons who devised instruments and operations to deal with deformity and disease. To begin with the application of their skills was limited by the problems of pain, shock, and infection. The turn of the nineteenth century saw a revolution in surgical practice, brought on by advances in anaesthesia, asepsis and anti-sepsis, and blood transfusion. These advances enabled a vast leap forward in surgical techniques so that sequentially the body cavities and their organs were exposed to the art and craft of surgery with increasingly dramatic outcomes. In the case of the heart, for example, valvotomy, followed by valve replacement, coronary artery grafting, and ultimately transplantation and even the implantation of an artificial heart, has prolonged the lives of those who otherwise would have died of their underlying disease.

Now as the century draws to a close, we are in the midst of a second surgical revolution, based on advances in imaging techniques, in particular fibre-optics and microchip cameras. These have led to awe inspiring, magnified images of the contents of the abdominal and thoracic cavities and the insides of many of the viscera. Projected on to large screens, sometimes with three-dimensional imagery, these developments, combined with the production of small instruments and miniaturised stapling machines, have allowed the development of minimal access and endoscopic surgery. We have to remember, however, that among the undoubted benefits of the first revolution, there were adverse sequelae. Inappropriate operations such as total colectomy for toxaemia, gastric freezing for haematemesis, colonic replacement of the removed stomach, and interval appendicectomy were all operations that subsequently were shown to be of no value or even of positive harm.

In 1988 the House of Lords Committee on Science and Technology called for the development of a more "evidence based" approach to medical practice. In particular, it recommended an assessment of the effectiveness and cost-effectiveness of existing and new technologies. Hence the Research and Development Directorate was established under the direction of Professor Sir Michael Peckham. As part of this initiative, the Standing Group on Health Technology was brought into being with the specific remit of assessing existing and new technologies. Enthusiasm for the potential of a new technology can lead to the evaluation of new procedures being bypassed, despite it being accepted since the days of John Hunter that innovations should be evaluated before being used on human beings. It requires strict discipline on the part of a surgeon presented with an exciting new technology to use that technology only within the context of a trial or a strict audit of outcome and complications. At a time when new technologies are appearing over the horizon at an increasing rate, it is important for surgeons to evaluate critically, not only the effectiveness, but also the cost-effectiveness and influence on quality of life of new technologies. It is our privilege to live in a time when advances in other sciences can be adapted for use in surgery. The sceptical surgeon is one who will always question whether a new technology is an advance on the existing technology, and if it is, whether it is cost-effective.

The Advisory Committee on Science and Technology, in its review of new surgical techniques, concluded that while new technologies could undoubtedly be of benefit, the possible adverse consequences, such as, for instance, the increased incidence of damage to the common bile duct in laparoscopic cholecystectomy, were such that new surgical technologies should be subjected to the same rigorous evaluation as drugs are subjected to by the Committee on Safety of Medicines. At the time of writing the process of establishing such a registry of new technologies is currently under way. It is planned that in the future the introduction of new technologies will be monitored through professional bodies such as the Royal College of Surgeons of England, and evaluated through a mechanism such as health technology assessment, supervised by the Standing Group on Health Technologies.

Of course, the story does not finish simply with the establishment of the safety and efficacy of new technique. It is a surgeon's professional responsibility to ensure that before embarking on a new technique he or she is adequately trained. Developments in simulation, ranging from the use of animal tissues, plastic materials, even through to virtual reality, now mean that it is possible for surgeons to train in laboratory based environments. The minimal access therapy training unit (MATTU) of the Royal College of Surgeons of England and the surgical workshops using anatomical prostheses (SWAP) mean that technique and experience can be established in a laboratory environment before the trainee surgeon works under supervision on human beings and before being allowed to practice independently.

My colleague, Tim Brown, and myself have produced this book at the request of British Medical Journal Publishing Group to illustrate the scope of minimal access surgery in the mid-1990s. We have tried to combine the enthusiasm of a talented young laparoscopic surgeon with the cautious approach of one charged with the responsibility for assessing the safety, effectiveness, and cost-effectiveness of new surgical techniques. We are well aware that some of the techniques described have yet to prove their superiority over existing techniques. We are impressed with the effectiveness with which standard surgical operations such as cholecystectomy can be carried out using laparoscopic methods, with the result that patients who would normally have stayed in hospital four to five days can go home in 48 hours and resume work in two weeks. At the same time we are aware that these benefits, that can apply to over 90% of patients undergoing, for example, cholecystectomy, are clouded by the undoubted, admittedly minute, increase in serious complications. We believe that the combination of enthusiastic adaptation of the many exciting new technologies currently being presented to surgeons, combined with a rigorous programme of appropriate evaluation, will lead to the safe introduction of new technologies, which will have as big an impact at the turn of this century as anaesthesia, asepsis and anti-sepsis, and blood transfusion had at the turn of the last.

Professor Sir Miles Irving
September 1995

Introduction

This book has been written to introduce the concepts and practices of minimal access surgery to surgeons in training, general practitioners, and medical students. It aims to cover the areas of laparoscopy, thoracoscopy, endoscopy in the head and neck, and arthroscopy. The widespread use of diagnostic and therapeutic endoscopy (gastroscopy, colonoscopy, ERCP) and techniques such as transurethral urology are outside the scope of this book.

Minimal access surgery has grown rapidly from a technique employed by the gynaecologist, urologist and a few enthusiastic general surgeons to being regularly used in general surgery, gynaecology, urology, thoracic surgery, orthopaedic surgery, and otolaryngology. The main impetus for this increase came from the development of laparoscopic cholecystectomy by Mouret in France in 1987, and by Reddick and Olsen in the USA. Laparoscopic cholecystectomy became accepted as the procedure of choice for cholecystectomy in many countries, and is now considered an essential part of training in general surgery.

General surgeons then began to apply the techniques they had learnt for laparoscopic cholecystectomy to other intraperitoneal operations, especially appendicectomy, inguinal hernia repair, and upper gastrointestinal surgery such as Nissen fundoplication and vagotomy. Surgery for malignant disease has been performed laparoscopically, although concerns with using such techniques for cancer (related to adequate tumour clearance and tumour implantation) mean that laparoscopic surgery for malignant disease should be performed only as part of a clinical trial. Urologists have used minimal access techniques to carry out transurethral surgery (on the prostate and on the bladder) for many years, and have developed techniques for lithotripsy and percutaneous lithotomy. They have also begun to employ laparoscopic techniques for renal surgery and more complicated intra-abdominal procedures.

Arthroscopy has been introduced in orthopaedic surgery, and now almost any major or medium sized joint may be examined using an arthroscope; therapeutic techniques are widely applied.

The developments in thoracic surgery have mirrored those in general surgery, and led to the possibility of intrathoracic surgery with a reduced likelihood of postoperative pain.

Otolaryngologists have also realised that the application of such techniques has a place in their surgical armamentarium, and this has been greatly benefited by the development of instruments and camera equipment.

Accompanying the advent of laparoscopic cholecystectomy has been a huge growth in the use of minimal access surgery in many branches of surgery—with a corresponding growth in journal articles, journals and books dedicated to issues related to minimal access surgery. Many of the books available cover the whole range of minimal access surgery, and are hence expensive; others cover a single operation (such as cholecystectomy), or a specialty (such as urology). The aim of this book is to introduce minimal access surgery across the spectrum of the surgical specialties at a level needed before sitting the CSIG examination. Therefore, procedures such as laparoscopic cholecystectomy are covered in some depth, but the chapters on gynaecology or urology are meant as a broad introduction, to lead an interested reader to one of the more specialised texts. Illustrations are used widely and written descriptions are accompanied by pictorial representations, which should improve understanding.

Acknowledgements

We wish to acknowledge the help and cooperation of many people in the preparation and publication of this book, especially in the production of the many illustrations.

The Medical Illustration Department of Wythenshawe Hospital in Manchester have reproduced many of the radiographs and instrument and "in-theatre" photographs. The Medical Illustration Departments at Hope Hospital and Manchester Royal Infirmary produced the "in-theatre" photographs in Chapters 7 and 9. The laparoscopic pictures reproduced in Chapters 6, 8, and 9 were taken using the Stryker 2-chip or 3-chip camera system, courtesy of Dean Sleigh and Brian Cleaver of Stryker, UK. The authors are very grateful for their help and cooperation in obtaining these pictures. The laparoscopic photographs in Chapter 7 were taken using Solos equipment distributed by Sigmacon on the Kodak Dry Process attached to the On-Call Photographer Office Based System from Sigmacon UK Ltd, Middlesex. The illustrations in Chapter 10 were produced by the Medical Illustration Department at Oldham Hospital, those in Chapter 11 were produced by the Medical Illustration Department at St Mary's Hospital, Manchester, those in Chapter 12 by the Medical Illustration Department at Leeds General Infirmary, and those in Chapter 14 by the Medical Illustration Department of Burton Hospital.

1 The history of laparoscopy

G Griffiths

Advances in diverse branches of medicine and physics have been required to develop laparoscopy and to bring it to the state where increasingly complex operative procedures are performed. These advances have taken place largely during the 20th century but it is only since 1987 that they have all come together to make modern operative laparoscopy possible. Techniques continue to evolve and the next decade will offer such attractions as stereoscopic vision and the use of virtual reality.

Greek and Roman physicians made the earliest attempts to view the interior of body cavities. Records from 400 BC show the physicians of Hippocrates' school using rectal and vaginal speculae. Similar instruments have been described from Pompeii (destroyed in AD 70) and from Babylon (around AD 500). It is assumed that these earliest endoscopes used daylight or a naked flame as illumination. These speculae have continued in use and in their development (Figure 1.1). Attempts at improving the light source probably started with the use of mirrors by Arabic physicians about AD 1000. Little progress was made for several hundreds of years, although in a report from 1587 a camera obscura was used to provide light to examine the nasal cavity. Lanterns were developed during the 18th century and in 1806 Bozzini used a tube to direct light from a lantern

to view the urethra and vagina. It is of interest, in light of the current laparoscopic expansion, that he was censured by the medical faculty of Vienna for being too inquisitive in performing this procedure. The next great advance came with Edison's invention of the light bulb in 1879: this not only revolutionised everyday life but also initiated the development of the light sources in use today.

Early attempts at laparoscopy

In the early part of the 20th century body orifices could be inspected with simple speculae and electric light. Three people lay claim to the development of laparoscopy. In 1901 Ott[1] described "ventroscopy", in which he inserted a speculum through an incision in the anterior abdominal wall and inspected the peritoneal cavity using light from a head mirror. Kelling[2] went one stage further, insufflating a dog's peritoneal cavity with air and viewing the contents with a cystoscope designed by Nitze in Berlin, 1877 (Figure 1.2). This technique was used by Jacobeus[4] in 1910 in his series of 115 examinations (abdomen and thorax) in 72 patients,

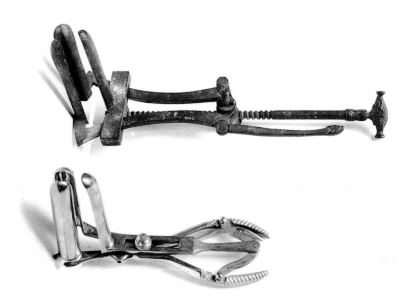

Figure 1.1 Rectal speculae: top, ancient; bottom, modern. Courtesy of the Wellcome Institute Library, London

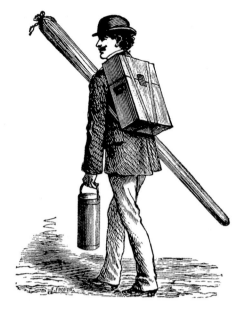

Figure 1.2 The Nitze–Leiter cystoscope of 1879, packed for transport. From Reference 3, courtesy of the Wellcome Institute Library, London

many of whom had ascites. He also described syphilis, tuberculosis, cirrhosis, and malignancy. With this report modern laparoscopy was born.

Instrument development

During the last 80 years every aspect of Jacobeus' procedure has been improved, with contributions from physics and surgery. A trocar for entering the abdominal cavity was developed by Nordentoeft[5] in 1912 and improved by Ordnoff in 1920,[6] when he introduced the pyramidal point used today. Before 1918 this trocar was used for initial entry into the peritoneal cavity, but in 1918 an insufflating needle was developed by Goetze[7] to make the establishment of a pneumoperitoneum much safer. Twenty years later, Veress[8] developed the blunt ended needle that remains in use today. Air was initially used for insufflation but CO_2, introduced in 1925 by Zollikofer,[9] was found to be safer than air due to its greater solubility. Around this time enthusiasm was so great for this new procedure that Short,[10] an English surgeon, advocated performing laparoscopy in the patient's home, adding interest to a domiciliary visit.

The development of therapeutic laparoscopy

By the 1930s the main use for laparoscopy was to diagnose intra-abdominal disease, particularly in the liver. This was made easier in 1929 with the introduction by Kalk[11] of an oblique viewing scope. Kalk was also the first to employ a second abdominal puncture to enable biopsies to be taken. Ruddock,[12] an American general physician,[13] published a series of 500 laparoscopies with 39 biopsies and attempted to enthuse his surgical colleagues by publishing in a surgical journal. General surgeons did not embrace laparoscopy, although Fervers,[14] a German surgeon, performed the first therapeutic laparoscopy in 1933 to carry out adhesiolysis.

The gynaecologists provided the main impetus to further developments. Bovie introduced diathermy in 1928, and it was used in the first laparoscopic sterilisations by Bosch in 1936[15] and Anderson in 1937.[16] In the same year Hope was the first to diagnose an ectopic pregnancy by laparoscopy.[17] In the 1940s laparoscopy continued to be developed in Europe, but in the USA culdoscopy became the preferred method of viewing the pelvis. Laparoscopy did not become more widely used in North America until the mid 1960s.

Insufflation

A prototype automatic insufflator was introduced by Fragenheim in the 1950s,[18] and the modern automatic insufflator developed during the 1960s and 1970s. This has progressed into the modern electronic instrument with high flow rates, gas extraction facilities and pressure alarms.

Light sources and lenses

Light was initially provided by siting a bulb either at the end of the laparoscope or close to it (Figure 1.3). The instrument consequently became very hot and burns were reported. In 1943 Fourestiere[19] was the first to effectively transmit light from an external source along a quartz rod to the laparoscope: this was the early cold light source. Fibreoptic cables, using the principle of total internal reflection, were first described in 1928 but they were not used to provide the convenient cold light source of today until 1957. Halogen bulbs in the 1970s further improved brightness.

Improving illumination has been, and remains, an important challenge. The invention of the rod lens

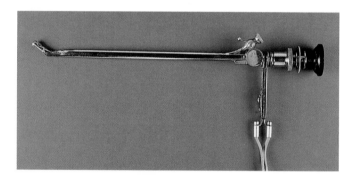

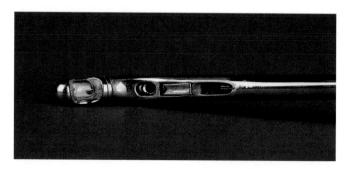

Figure 1.3 Example of a cystoscope that would allow vision and instrumentation. Note the position of the light bulb at the tip (bottom picture) (figures kindly supplied by MWM Lau)

system by Hopkins in 1953 was an important advance in making a brighter image, but it was not used clinically until 1967. In a rod lens system most of the light in the laparoscope passes through glass. The lenses are small pockets of air between appropriately shaped glass rods. Coating the glass surfaces with magnesium fluoride evaporated in a vacuum reduces reflections and further improves the image.

Modern developments

Modern therapeutic laparoscopy became possible in the early 1980s, when the silicon chip television camera was invented. This enabled a small lightweight attachment on the end of the laparoscope to be used to provide an image magnified on a screen. The surgeon's hands were free to operate and the laparoscope could be manipulated by an assistant. The first laparoscopic cholecystectomy was performed by Mouret in 1987.[20] Early series were reported by Reddick[21] in 1989 and Dubois[22] in 1990. Laser dissection was used in several of these early series; it was first used laparoscopically by Bruhat[23] for dividing adhesions and destroying endometriotic deposits. Blunt dissection and diathermy remain very popular methods of laparoscopic dissection. The number of centres offering laparoscopic surgery has risen rapidly since 1990, including most, if not all, district general hospitals. New operative techniques are being developed and laparoscopy is finding a place in gastric surgery, hernia repair, appendicectomy and colonic surgery.

The history of laparoscopy illustrates how a clinical impetus leads to the development and application of new techniques. Continued public and professional demands for minimal access surgery will drive further advances and laparoscopy in the 21st century will differ as much from today's technique as this differs from Ott's original ventroscopy.

1 von Ott D. Die direkte Beleuchtung der Bauchhohle, der Harnblase, des Dickdarms und des Uterus zu diagnostischen Zwecken. *Rev Med Tcheque* (Prague) 1901;2:27.
2 Kelling G. Uber Oesophagoskopie, Gastroskopie und Colioskopie. *Munch Wschr* 1902;49:21–24.
3 Cotwell HA. *An essay on the history of electrotherapy and diagnosis.* London, 1992;119.
4 Jacobeus H. Uber Laparo- und Thoracoskopie. *Beitrage zur Klinik Tuberk* 1912;25:183–254.
5 Nordentoeft S. Uber Endoskopie geschlossener Kavitaten mittels meines Trokar-Endoskopes. *Verhandlungen der Deutchen Gesellschaft fur Gynakologie* 1912;41:78–81.
6 Easkin TA, Isobe JH, Mathews JL, Winchester SB, Smith RJ. Laparoscopy and the general surgeon. *Surg Clin North Am* 1991;71:1085–97.
7 Goetze O. Die Rontgendiagnostik bei gasgefullter Bauchhole eine neue Methode. *Munch Med Wschr* 1918;65:1275–80.
8 Veress J. Ein Neues Instrument zur Ausfuhrung von Brust – oder Bauchpunktionen und Pneumothoraxbehandlung. *Dtsch Med Wschr* 1938;64:1480–1.
9 Zollikofer R. Zur Laparsokopie. *Schweiz Med Wschr* 1924;5:264–5.
10 Short R. The uses of coelioscopy. *BMJ* 1925;2:254–5.
11 Kalk H. Erfahrungen mit der Laparoskopie. *Z Klin Med* 1929;111:303.
12 Ruddock JC. Peritoneoscopy. *Surg Gynecol Obstet* 1937;65:623.
13 Stellato TA. History of laparoscopic surgery. *Surg Clin North Am* 1992;72:997–1002.
14 Fervers C. Die Laparoskopie mit dem Cystoskope. Ein Beitrag zur Vereinfachung der Tachnik und zur endoskopischen Strangdurchtrennung in der Bauchole. *Med Klin* 1933;29:1042–5.
15 Bosch PF. *Laparoskopische sterilization.* Schweizerische Zeitschrift fur Krankenhaus und Anstaltswesen, 1936.
16 Anderson ET. Peritoneoscopy. *Am J Surg* 1937;35:136–9.
17 Hope R. The differential diagnosis of ectopic pregnancy by peritoneoscopy. *Surg Gynecol Obstet* 1937;64:229–34.
18 Fragenheim H. In: Gordon AG, Lewis, BV (eds). *History of endoscopy.* London: Chapman and Hall, 1988.
19 Fourestiere M, Gladu A, Vulmiere J. La peritoneoscopie. *Presse Medicale* 1943;5:46–7.
20 Mouret G. From the first laparoscopic cholecystectomy to the frontiers of laparoscopic surgery: the future perspective. *Dig Surg* 1991;8:12–5.
21 Reddick E, Olsen D. Laparoscopic laser cholecystectomy: a comparison with mini-laparotomy cholecystectomy. *Surg Endosc* 1989;3:131.
22 Dubois F, Card P, Berthelot G *et al.* Coelioscopic cholecystectomy: preliminary report of thirty six cases. *Ann Surg* 1990;211:60.
23 Bruhat MA, Mage G, Manhes M. Use of CO_2 laser by laparoscopy. In: Kaplan I (ed) *Laser surgery III. Proceedings of the third international congress on laser surgery.* Tel Aviv: Jerusalem Press, 1979:275.

2 Equipment for laparoscopic surgery

M M Mughal

Good equipment is more important in laparoscopic surgery than in open surgery. Unsatisfactory insufflation, poor views and inappropriate grasping instruments can make it impossible to perform an otherwise feasible laparoscopic procedure. The range and variety of instruments have increased rapidly in the last few years to keep pace with an increasing variety of laparoscopic procedures. This chapter will cover basic laparoscopic equipment used to perform common laparoscopic procedures such as cholecystectomy, appendicectomy, hernia repair, vagotomy, and fundoplication. Special instruments for other procedures can be added to the set if required for more specialised procedures. Important as it is to have good equipment, the surgeon, assistants, theatre nurses, and technicians (that is, all those who will have some role in setting up and operating the equipment) must know how each device and instrument works. Disposable instruments must not be sterilised and reused unless this is allowed by the manufacturer. Instruments for open surgery, including vascular clamps and sutures, must always be available in case the laparoscopic procedure has to be abandoned.

Equipment for pneumoperitoneum

Creating a pneumoperitoneum

This is usually carried out "blindly" using the Veress needle (Figure 2.1). This is available in different lengths

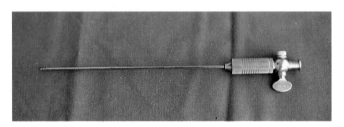

Figure 2.1 Veress needle

and it is useful to have one or two longer needles in addition to the standard sizes, for use in obese patients. The reusable needle tip is prone to blunting after extensive use and should be checked before insertion. Correct assembly of the needle includes the use of a compatible obturator. A standard length obturator

inserted into a long needle will not spring out beyond the needle tip resulting in possible damage to viscera. The spring action must be checked to ensure it works properly.

The use of a Veress needle in an extensively scarred abdomen may be hazardous but this problem can be overcome by using the open technique to insert the trocar. A small incision is made at the chosen site and the dissection deepened through the layers of the abdomen. The peritoneum should be free of adhesions and opened under direct vision. The Hassan cannula, designed for use in such circumstances, may then be inserted into the peritoneal cavity and secured by a purse string suture to provide a gas seal. It is usually possible to secure a standard 10 mm cannula in place with properly placed purse string sutures.

Maintaining the pneumoperitoneum

A good insufflator (Figure 2.2) is essential for procedures requiring several ports and constant

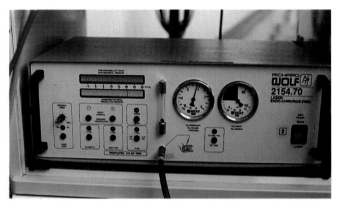

Figure 2.2 Equipment for insufflation, showing the tubing that connects with the patient

exchange of instruments which, with the use of suction, leads to loss of gas. For most abdominal procedures the gas used is carbon dioxide at a pressure of 15 mmHg. It should be possible to select both the pressure and the flow rate and the insufflator should have an indicator to warn if the intra-abdominal pressure exceeds the preset pressure. It is also useful to have a display of pressure in the gas reservoir so that if the supply is running low it can be replaced at an appropriate time during a procedure. Most insufflators have three flow settings: low flow (usually 1 l/min), high flow (10 l/min), and automatic to maintain the pneumoperitoneum by replenishing gas lost during exchange of instruments. The insufflator should be placed where the surgeon can easily see its display panel.

Access ports

Abdominal procedures rarely require the use of more than five ports, and usually four are sufficient. Ports are available in various sizes to match the different sized instruments and may be disposable or reusable (Figure 2.3). Straight scissors, graspers and dissectors usually go through a 5 mm port and telescopes through one of

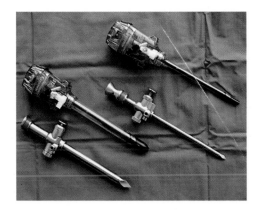

Figure 2.3 Disposable and reusable ports for introduction into the peritoneum. Both 5 mm and 10 mm ports are shown

10 mm. Stapling instruments and curved needles may require larger ports, usually 12 mm. The larger ports can be used for instruments with a smaller diameter by using appropriate reducers.

The choice between disposable and reusable ports is largely based on personal preference and financial constraints. Disposable ports are more expensive than reusable ports but, because the trocar is very sharp, are easier to insert. Many disposable ports now available have a safety shield, which springs out to cover the trocar point once it is inside the body cavity, and are therefore theoretically safer than reusable ports. Radiolucent disposable ports are advantageous when operative cholangiography is planned. Because disposable ports do not have trumpet valves, they are less likely than the non-disposable ones to damage any instruments inserted through them. Some surgeons use a mixture of disposable and reusable ports, using a shielded non-disposable device to establish the first "blind" port after establishing a pneumoperitoneum. Non-disposable ports must be kept in good working order by ensuring that they are cleaned and assembled properly, that the trumpet valves work smoothly, and that the gas seal washers are intact and effective.

Imaging equipment

Telescopes

A good telescope and camera (Figure 2.4) are an essential part of the laparoscopic armamentarium. Telescopes generally come in two sizes, 5 or 10 mm, and with several viewing angles. The 10 mm telescopes give

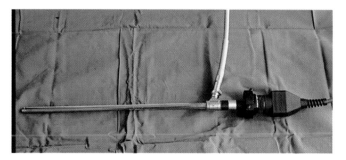

Figure 2.4 Laparoscope and attached camera

better views and carry more light for illumination than the smaller ones, and are therefore commonly used for operative procedures. A viewing angle of 0° denotes a forward viewing telescope, which is used for most procedures. A 30° telescope may be used for looking down, sideways or up at the operative field. It is useful for looking up during a hernia repair and for looking down when working at the diaphragmatic hiatus or the bile duct. Ideally, a 0° and a 30° telescope should be available on each set.

Light source, camera and monitors

The light source (Figure 2.5a) for most imaging systems forms part of a package made up of the camera,

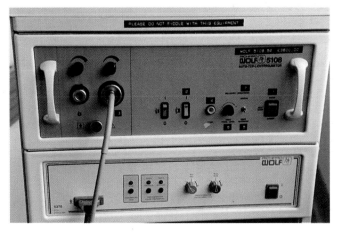

(a)

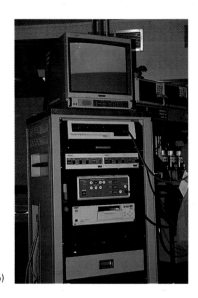

(b)

Figure 2.5 (a) Close up view of light source and camera connection. (b) Trolley holding monitor, camera and light source, insufflator, and video processor

video processor and television monitor (Figure 2.5b). In most modern systems the light source is linked to the video processor, which automatically controls light intensity by a feedback mechanism through the camera. This reduces glare and ensures uniform illumination of the operative field. With many systems the "white balance" must be reset each time the system is switched on in order to obtain true colours. The "white balance" should be set only after the light source has warmed up, usually a matter of 2–3 min after switching it on. The white balance is affected by the optics of the telescope and may need to be reset when telescopes are exchanged. A spare bulb for the light source must always be available, and it is imperative that the staff responsible for this know how to replace a bulb if necessary.

A variety of cameras is available for laparoscopic work. The original two chip cameras are being replaced with three chip cameras capable of very high resolution. Telescope-less cameras are also available, the camera chip being mounted at the end of a rod containing fibre bundles to carry light: as there is no optical interface between the object and camera (as in the usual telescope–camera assembly) the views obtained with such cameras are extremely good. Cameras are very delicate and easily damaged. If the camera housing and plug are not adequately protected during wet sterilisation, fluid may seep in—with dire consequences. To avoid such problems most surgeons no longer sterilise the camera and lead; instead slipping the unit into a sterile plastic sleeve, which is pulled over the telescope once the camera has been connected. If towel clips are used to secure cables and tubes particular care must be taken not to damage the camera lead.

Monitors should be of a resolution to match that of the camera system. One or two monitors may be used, depending on the procedure and how the surgeon deploys the assistants round the operating table. Video processors provide split screen facilities to display a second image if necessary—for instance when using two cameras in exploration of the common bile duct, or during laparoscopic ultrasound examination.

All the electronic and electrical equipment should ideally be mounted neatly and securely in one cabinet, with all the interconnections secure but accessible from the back of the cabinet. Then only one power supply is necessary to the cabinet, feeding all the items within it.

Instruments

Dissection, grasping and cutting

Curved and straight dissectors, as used in open surgery, preferably with diathermy attachment to allow grasping and coagulation of small vessels, are useful. Similarly, both curved and straight scissors should be available. Straight scissors are used for dividing a structure such as the cystic duct between clips, where separation between the clips may not be sufficient to allow the use of curved scissors, but curved scissors with rotatable tips are invaluable for general dissection (Figure 2.6). Most scissors have a diathermy attachment, extremely useful for coagulating small vessels encountered during dissection. It should be noted, however, that applying a diathermy current through the cutting edges of the scissors will blunt them. The diathermy hook (Figure 2.7a) is an extremely

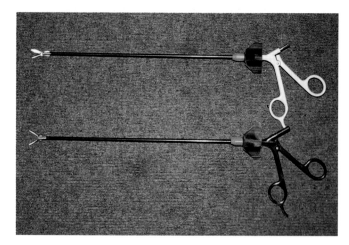

Figure 2.6 Curved scissors (top) and curved dissecting forceps (bottom) with rotatable tips

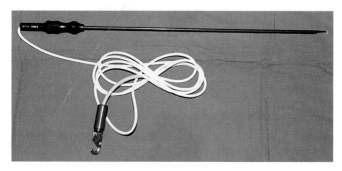

(a)

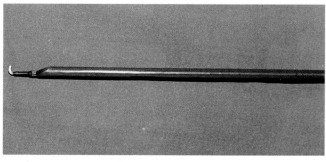

(b)

Figure 2.7 Hook diathermy with attached lead (a), and close up showing J shaped hook (b)

versatile piece of equipment that can be used as a dissecting, coagulating, and cutting instrument. It is available in a variety of shapes and sizes. The small J shaped hook, mounted at the end of a doubly insulated rod with only the hook exposed (Figure 2.7b), is very useful, as its use brings no risk of inadvertent diathermy to an adjacent structure from a long uninsulated straight limb of the J.

Both atraumatic and heavy graspers should be available. Light graspers and laparoscopic Babcock forceps (Figure 2.8) are useful for holding bowel but heavy graspers (Figure 2.9) are necessary for securing a good grip on a thick walled gall bladder. Several good tools are available for this; the three pronged bulldog forceps not only grasps the gall bladder well, but can also be used to grasp large stones. A general laparoscopic set should contain curved and straight

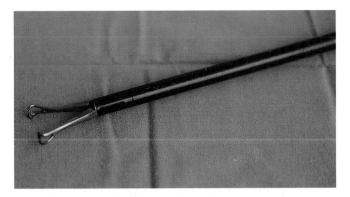

Figure 2.8 Laparoscopic Babcock forceps

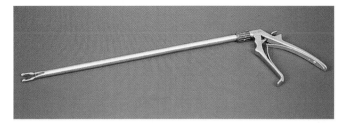

(a)

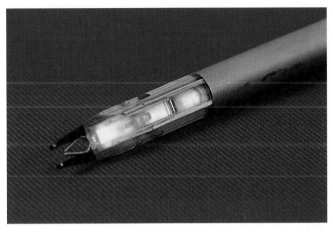

(b)

Figure 2.10 Reusable clip applier (a) and distal tip of multifire disposable applicator (b)

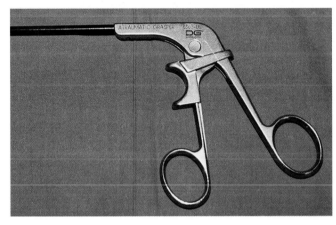

(a)

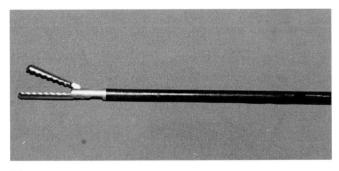

(b)

Figure 2.9 Grasping forceps for the gall bladder, showing (a) the device for fixing the handle and (b) a close up of the grasping end

dissectors, curved and straight scissors, Babcock type forceps, two heavy graspers, and one bulldog type grasper.

Haemostasis

Usually haemostasis is achieved by applying monopolar diathermy through scissors, dissecting forceps, or hook. Bipolar diathermy may also be used, but only through an instrument such as the grasper, in which the jaws act as the electrodes. Although it is, in theory, safer than monopolar diathermy, bipolar diathermy can be applied only through grasping instruments and the coagulated tissue tends to stick firmly to the jaws of the grasping instrument. In practice, therefore, bipolar diathermy is of limited use. Larger vessels are occluded with clips, using a reusable

clip applier (Figure 2.10a) or a multifire disposable applicator (Figure 2.10b).

Laser light may also be used for coagulation and cutting but in most situations has very little advantage over diathermy. Laser is therefore an optional, rather than an essential, piece of equipment.

Larger pedicles may be ligated or transected with the linear stapler, which cuts between two straight staple lines, each line being made of two staggered rows of staples. Pressure can be applied to a bleeding point in the same way as in open surgery by grasping a pledget firmly with a grasper passed through a 10–5 mm reducer, inserted through a 10 mm port.

Suturing and stapling

Suturing requires appropriate needles and needle holders. Ski shaped needles have been specially developed for laparoscopic surgery for easy insertion through 10 mm ports. The straight part of such a needle has a rectangular cross section so that the needle can not twist round its long axis once it is firmly grasped. Ordinary curved needles may, however, be used for laparoscopic surgery, although the curve of the needle may need to be reduced before it can be inserted through a port of 10 or 12 mm. A good needle holder is essential for laparoscopic suturing (Figure 2.11).

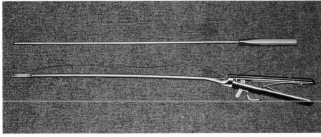

Figure 2.11 Needle holder (bottom) and knot pusher (top)

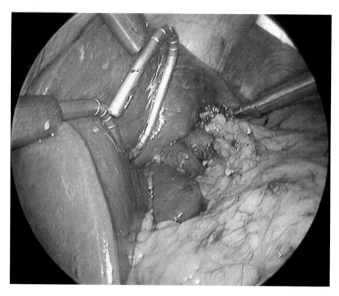

Figure 2.12 Adjustable retractor, showing the triangle shape that may be achieved when retracting the liver

Once the suture has been placed the knot can be tied inside or outside the body cavity and seated using a knot pusher. Preformed endoloops based on the Roeder slip knot are also available for ligating pedicles. Staplers are available to secure mesh to the abdominal wall in hernia repair, and linear staplers may be used for anastomosing two pieces of bowel in the same way as in open surgery.

Retractors

Good laparoscopic retractors have become available only recently, and have greatly added to the scope of laparoscopic surgery. A common design, useful for retracting the liver, opens into a fan. The rod and wire retractor is a particularly ingenious, robust and versatile device. It is inserted through a 6 mm port. By turning a screw on the handle of the retractor, the wire passing through the rod is tightened and the shape of the tip changes. The retractor is available to form a variety of shapes such as a triangle (Figure 2.12) (for retracting the omentum or liver), and to curve on an angle (for example, for getting round the oesophagus).

Miscellaneous tools

Of these the most important is undoubtedly the suction irrigator, most of which are 5 mm in diameter. Irrigation is more effective under pressure and pumps are available for this purpose, but using a pressure bag around a bag of irrigation fluid works quite well. The 5 mm sucker is prone to blockage with debris and clots, and a 10 mm suction aspirator is available to overcome this problem. A variety of bags is available for extracting extruded stones, entire gall bladder or a detached, inflamed appendix. Devices are also available to stretch a port site for easier extraction of the large, packed gall bladder.

Summary

1. The basic set for laparoscopic surgery requires only a few essential good quality instruments, and may be added to as required.
2. Two complete sets of cables, tubes, telescopes, ports, and instruments allow backup for instrument failure and the next procedure to begin without delay.
3. Everyone concerned should know how the equipment works, and how to clean and maintain it.
4. Disposable equipment should not be reused unless otherwise instructed by the manufacturer.
5. A set of instruments for open surgery should be readily available in case the laparoscopic operation has to be abandoned.

3 Laparoscopic techniques

Timothy H Brown

The introduction of endoscopic surgery ensured a need to learn and develop techniques for use laparoscopically, which are not used in open surgery. These techniques are applicable whether the surgery involves the gall bladder, the uterus, the appendix, the lung, or any other organs, but they vary substantially from techniques used in open surgery. The main reasons for different techniques being needed in laparoscopic surgery are:

- Increased distance between hands and tissue
- Rigid instruments functioning as levers
- Video vision, not direct vision
- Two dimensional, not three dimensional vision
- Inability to palpate

The surgeon must adjust to operating without being able to directly visualise the ends of the instruments, operating in two rather than three dimensions, and being unable to palpate tissues to assess what they are, their strength, or their relative position.

Insufflation

For laparoscopic surgery it is necessary to introduce CO_2 into the peritoneal cavity. This is achieved via a Veress needle (see Chapter 2) introduced through a subumbilical transverse or midline incision. Many surgeons elevate the abdominal wall by grasping each side of the umbilicus, or just below the umbilicus, and introduce the needle while it is elevated. It may be easier to incise down to the anterior rectus, then grasp this with Allis forceps and elevate the abdominal wall. The recti and the peritoneum are lifted and a suture placed each side of the midline used to elevate the recti (later

these can be ligated to close the port defect). The Veress needle, and subsequently the 10 mm port, are then introduced with relative ease (Figure 3.1). Care must be taken to suture the rectus sheath and not the fascia or fat, as retracting on these structures will increase the difficulty of introducing the needle. The Veress needle is carefully introduced, ensuring that it is not plunged into an intraperitoneal structure; the surgeon should be able to feel it pass through the two layers of the abdominal wall. Saline is introduced down the needle and aspirated to ensure that the needle is not placed in the bowel, and a drop of saline is left on the tip of the needle (Figure 3.2). The sutures are elevated and if the end of the needle is correctly placed the drop of saline will be sucked into the peritoneal cavity. When this occurs insufflation of the peritoneal cavity with CO_2 may safely be commenced at 1 l/min and then at 4 l/min to a maximum of 15 mmHg. A high pressure at this stage may indicate that the needle is placed extraperitoneally or into adhesions.

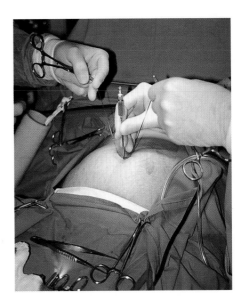

Figure 3.1 Introduction of Veress needle demonstrating elevation of the abdominal wall using sutures placed in the rectus sheath

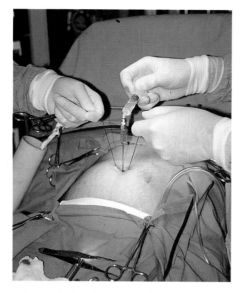

Figure 3.2 Droplet test on Veress needle

Dissection

Perhaps the most common of the techniques used in endoscopic surgery is dissection. A variety of endoscopic dissecting forceps is available but the designs are similar: a long straight instrument with a curved, toothed end that can be opened and closed to separate tissues, to grasp tissue and strip it away, to separate tissue with blunt dissection (Figure 3.3), to hold tissue to allow ligation or diathermy, or to help in some of the more complicated techniques. Recent improvements in the design of instruments include the facility of diathermy along the forceps, which allows control of haemorrhage with one instrument rather than two.

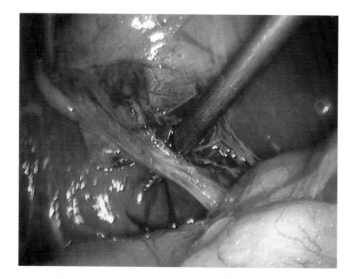

Figure 3.3 Separation of tissue using blunt dissecting forceps

Scissors may be used for dissection to allow the surgeon to dissect or divide without exchanging instruments. Hydrodissection using an irrigation device connected to a pressure bag may also be used to separate planes by blunt, non-haemorrhagic dissection. This technique is particularly useful for injecting saline between the gall bladder and liver bed before separating them.

Ligation

Haemorrhage can be controlled by diathermy but other techniques enable vessels, ducts or other structures to be ligated.

The structure may be clipped; there are instruments specifically constructed to enable such a manoeuvre (Figure 3.4). Clip appliers may be placed through a 10 mm port and are supplied in reusable, reloadable or disposable forms. The clips generally used are made of titanium, although dissolvable clips are now available. Such clips are used on the cystic duct and cystic artery during laparoscopic cholecystectomy. To place the clips successfully requires a two handed technique; the instrument in the left hand holds the vessel or duct to be clipped and the clip applier is held in the right hand. If structures need to be double clipped and divided a multifire clip applier is of most use, particularly for ligating and dividing the short gastric vessels when mobilising the fundus of the stomach before performing the wrap of a Nissen fundoplication.

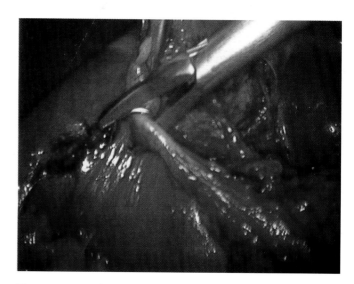

Figure 3.4 Clip placed using clip applier

A more complicated ligation technique involves the placement of a pretied loop of suture material bearing a Roeder knot, known as an Endoloop or Ethibinder (Ethicon Endosurgery, Edinburgh) (Figure 3.5). This device is back loaded into a reducing port to conceal the loose loop, the reducing port is placed into a 10 mm port, and the loop introduced into the peritoneal cavity. The tissue to be ligated, for example the appendix, is then manipulated towards the loose loop and grasping forceps placed through the loop to grasp the tissue and pull it back through the loop. With the loop around the base of the tissue the external end of the loop is snapped and the knot tightened by holding the suture and pushing on the plastic sheath. Advancement of the knot is observed via the endoscope and the knot is manipulated until it is fully tightened around the area to be ligated (Figure 3.6). The external ligature is divided and the pusher withdrawn, a pair of scissors introduced, and the suture divided near the tightened knot.

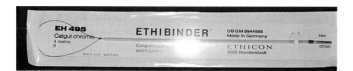

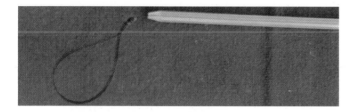

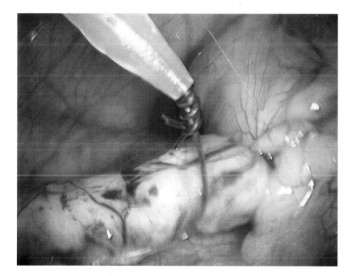

Figure 3.6 Loop being tightened around the appendix

Knots may be tied extracorporeally[1] or intracorporeally. Extracorporeal suturing requires the suture to be grasped by the needle holder, just beyond the needle hub, after it has passed through the tissues and pulled back up the port. Once outside, the first throw is placed and the throw pushed down the port and tightened using a knot pusher (of which several designs are available). This procedure is repeated until three or four alternating throws have been placed, and the surgeon is sure that the knot is secure. The long lengths of the suture may then be divided. A second method for extracorporeal suturing is known as the Roeder knot. This knot is tied outside the abdomen and slipped down a port into the peritoneum where it is closed by advancing until tight. The principle used is that of a slip knot, which locks as it is tightened.

For intracorporeal suturing the trailing end of the suture needs to be relatively short and easily visible in the field of view. The needle is grasped at its hub by the grasper in the left hand and the needle holder is wound around the needle three times. The surgeon grasps the short end of the suture with the needle holder and pulls it through the loops of suture. The next throw is placed in the opposite direction using the same technique, so that the knot locks. Further throws may be placed to ensure that the knot is tight and secure. It can be difficult to gauge the tightness of the knots when tied like this, and the technique is complicated to learn. However, once mastered, this technique may be used in a number of different situations.

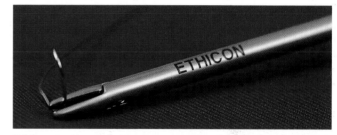

Figure 3.7 Needle holder demonstrating tip for grasping needle

Suturing

Suturing is one of the more complex techniques used in laparoscopic surgery. It is rarely required for laparoscopic cholecystectomy, appendicectomy or hernia repair but it is an essential part of the procedure for laparoscopic Nissen fundoplication and for other advanced procedures. Needle holders are available from several manufacturers but the best design involves a ratcheted handle and a ribbed grasping end, which will tend to rotate the needle to 90° to the needle holder on closing (Figure 3.7). The best needle for most applications is a small curved needle, rather than the ski needle introduced for laparoscopic use. The needle needs a shallow enough curve to allow it to pass down a 10 mm port, and is introduced by grasping the suture proximal to the junction with the needle and passing it down the port. Once the needle is visible it is grasped by an instrument in the left hand and held in the correct orientation for the needle holder to grasp and suture. The needle is driven through the tissue (Figure 3.8) or the tissue is pushed over the needle, and once it is visible through the tissue the surgeon uses the grasper in the left hand to pull the needle through the tissue and hold it until it can be regrasped by the needle holder.

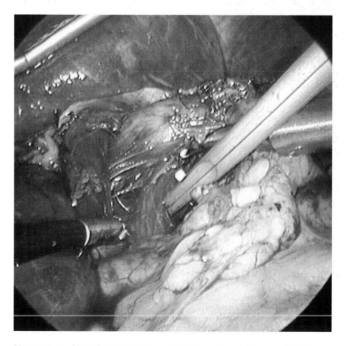

Figure 3.8 Needle placed through tissue, the left crus at the hiatus

Extraction

Successful laparoscopic surgery also requires the removed tissue to be extracted. This is usually the gall bladder, but recent developments have allowed larger amounts of tissue to be removed, some of which may be malignant. A relatively collapsed gall bladder or appendix (Figure 3.9) can be extracted through the port.

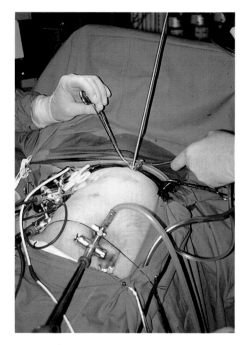

Figure 3.10 Gall bladder emptied at the skin surface using suction

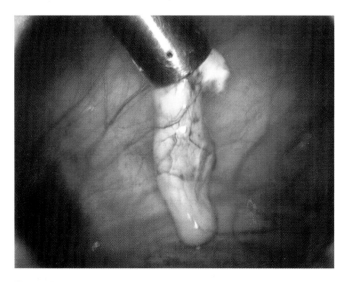

Figure 3.9 Appendix extracted via port

If this is not possible the gall bladder may be pulled to the abdominal skin through the port, the port removed and the gall bladder emptied by suction (Figure 3.10) and/or stone extraction and removed without spilling its contents into the peritoneal cavity. If the surgeon is concerned that the gall bladder may rupture during extraction, or if the gall bladder has been damaged during its resection, then it should be placed in a bag before removal. The "Bert" bag (Bag for the Endoscopic Retrieval of Tissue, Vernon Carus Ltd, Preston, UK) is the most widely available bag for this technique (Figure 3.11). It is designed so that it will not split on removal. The gall bladder may be manipulated into this bag, pulled to the skin surface and removed in the bag. Alternatively, the bag can be opened and the gall bladder aspirated, or the stones removed, before attempting to extract the gall bladder.

If malignant tissue is to be removed a hole larger than the tissue must be made, as malignant tissue should not be allowed contact with the skin, because of the risk of implantation of cells. It is wise under these circumstances to place the tissue in an impermeable bag before extraction.

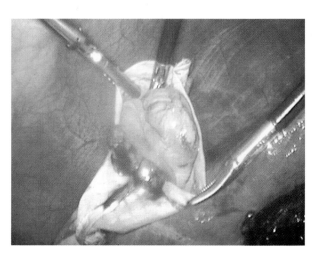

Figure 3.11 Gall bladder placed in Bert bag

Acknowledgements

The author is grateful to Stryker UK for the equipment used for the intraoperative illustrations (Figures 3, 4, 6, 8 and 9), and to Ethicon Endosurgery for Figure 7.

1 Kennedy JS. A technique for extracorporeal suturing. *J Laparoendosc Surg* 1992;2:269–72.

4 Training in laparoscopic surgery

Nigel A Scott

Laparoscopic surgery requires training

As with all surgical apprenticeships, training for laparoscopic surgery should involve a combination of theoretical teaching, practical instruction using simulation, and supervised operative experience. Training schemes are not foreign to surgical practice, and have evolved informally in areas such as gastrointestinal endoscopy. However, the immense potential of laparoscopic surgery to inflict harm when wielded by the untrained surgeon mandates a structured formal training approach.

The trainee should have completed basic surgical training and be familiar with the assessment and perioperative management of conditions that require laparoscopic surgery, including conventional surgical alternatives. Formal training in laparoscopic operative surgery should form part of any higher surgical training. At present, consultants who were in post when laparoscopic surgery was introduced also need training,[1] because many have taken up laparoscopic surgery without adequate training, and the Royal College of Surgeons of England have now issued guidelines for such training.

Stages in training

- Familiarisation with equipment
- Practical instruction with simulation
- Supervised operative training
- Assessment by an independent laparoscopic surgeon

Three distinct stages in the training for laparoscopic surgery take the surgeon through familiarisation with the supportive and operative equipment, practical instruction using simulation and on to supervised operative training. A fourth stage, assessment by an independent laparoscopic surgeon, could be added. However, such is the novelty of this surgery that the technique of even the trained laparoscopic surgeon will be refined by further equipment familiarisation, simulator experience, and (where necessary) further supervised operative experience.

Familiarisation with equipment

A fundamental departure of laparoscopic surgery from conventional surgery is in the use and dependence of the surgeon on complex equipment.

Camera, monitors and insufflator

The major capital cost of establishing laparoscopic surgery lies in the purchase of monitors, a laparoscopic camera, a light source, an insufflator, and a diathermy machine (occasionally a laser source is used) (Figure 4.1). It is important that the trainee laparoscopic surgeon becomes thoroughly acquainted with all aspects

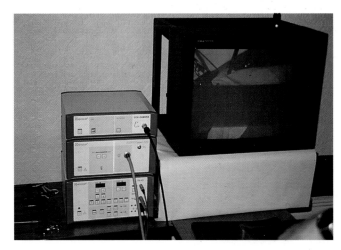

Figure 4.1 Monitor, light source and camera unit

of this equipment and its use. The surgeon should help to set up the monitors, check the carbon dioxide supply to the insufflator and ensure that the camera and light system is working. This practice is analogous to the checks that an anaesthetist performs before commencing anaesthesia.

Manipulative and operative equipment

Before starting any form of laparoscopic surgery the trainee must become familiar with the trocars, needles, and operative equipment introduced into the body and used to grasp, pull, and cut tissues. Early in their training, trainees should handle the laparoscopic instruments before and after a laparoscopic operation. This should allow them to recognise the instruments (dissecting forceps, diathermy hooks, graspers, and suction cannulas) and become familiar with their action before intraoperative use.

Operative simulation

The fine control of tissue manipulation with an instrument 30 cm long is unlike any other conventional daily activity. This means that the trainee surgeon must learn the feel and look of laparoscopic surgery in a simulator before progressing to supervised operative experience. Laparoscopic simulators fall into three main groups:

- plastic see through box;
- fully equipped station with animal organ in jig;
- anaesthetised animal.

Plastic box

This is ideal for use in the classroom, the on-call room, or the living room at home. With an array of cleaned disposable equipment it is possible to carry out a range of basic laparoscopic manoeuvres, beginning with port insertion through the soft plastic cover and followed by instrument insertion into the cavity of the box. A camera is not necessary, as all manoeuvres are viewed directly through the clear plastic cover.

Foam rubber may be used to represent tissue and can be grasped, clipped, and cut. Small balloons partly filled with liquid may be fixed in the simulator to represent a gall bladder and cystic duct. The cystic duct can be occluded with clips and divided. Extracorporeal and intracorporeal knotting can also be practised.

The plastic box simulator is not for detailed rehearsal of specific operations, but allows repeated practice of laparoscopic instrument manipulation in an informal fashion.

Fully equipped station

A fully equipped station (Figure 4.2) is usually available for simulation of laparoscopic surgery only

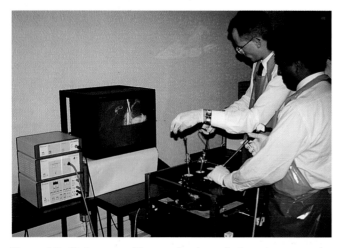

Figure 4.2 Trainees working on simulator during a laparoscopic course

within the context of a laparoscopic course. Access to this level of simulation allows further use and understanding of the camera, monitors, insufflator and diathermy machine in a controlled setting. It is possible to practice manipulation of foam rubber and balloon models of laparoscopic surgery.

An added advantage of the fully equipped station is the ability to practice tissue dissection on animal organs fixed into the purpose built jigs (Figure 4.3).

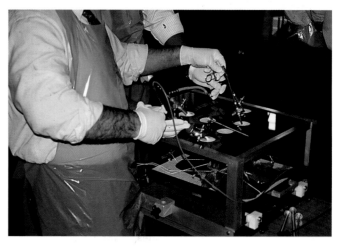

Figure 4.3 Trainees working on animal liver in the simulator

For example, sheep livers form a suitable model for rehearsing the basics of laparoscopic cholecystectomy. Storage and disposal of this offal must satisfy health and safety regulations, and it is crucial to ensure that the livers are provided with the gall bladder and biliary tree still attached. The animal liver is tied into the jig and a full laparoscopic cholecystectomy rehearsed. Four ports are introduced, the fundus of the gall bladder is grasped and dissection is performed to demonstrate the cystic duct and cystic artery. These structures can be clipped and divided and the gall bladder removed. In a single session two trainees acting alternately as surgeon and camera operator/assistant should be able to perform three simulated laparoscopic cholecystectomies each. The use of lengths of small bowel with attached mesentery can also allow simulated appendicectomy to be performed.

Involvement of the nursing staff in a fully simulated laparoscopic procedure is also of great benefit. New theatre nursing staff may have little opportunity to see and understand how laparoscopic equipment functions without the pressures of daily work. Night staff in theatres are notoriously isolated from developments in laparoscopic surgery, and their inclusion on a laparoscopic course is of considerable benefit to all concerned.

Courses for training in laparoscopic surgery are arranged locally, nationally or internationally. The Wolfson Foundation has established three training centres for such courses: the Minimal Access Therapy Training Unit (Figure 4.4) at the Royal College of Surgeons of England in London (MATTU), the Leeds Institute for Minimally Invasive Surgery (LIMIT), and the Minimal Access Therapy Training Unit, Scotland, in Dundee (MATTUS) Each of these centres runs training courses (Figure 4.5). The purpose of these centres is to teach consultant surgeons and trainees basic and advanced laparoscopic surgery. There are also privately run centres in Dublin, Paris and Hamburg, where training is available for some of the more complicated laparoscopic procedures. The centres in Europe also provide experience in laparoscopic procedures on the anaesthetised animal, which is not allowed in the UK.

Anaesthetised animal

The anaesthetised animal, which is killed immediately after the surgical procedure, clearly provides a

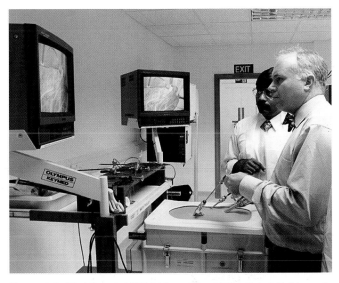

Figure 4.4 Training at MATTU (courtesy of the Royal College of Surgeons of England)

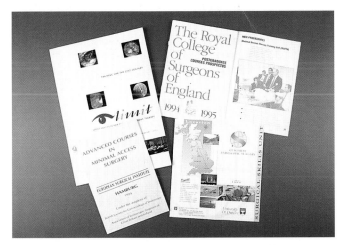

Figure 4.5 Brochures for the various centres that offer training in laparoscopic techniques

laparoscopic simulation that is much closer to that of operating on a patient than simulators.[2] The feel of the introduction of a pneumoperitoneum and port insertion is identical to that experienced in a human patient. Tissue handling and the control of bleeding using diathermy and clips is clearly much closer to reality than any other form of simulation. In addition, specific complex surgical procedures such as rectopexy or Nissen fundoplication can be both taught and rehearsed in the anaesthetised animal.

This type of surgical training is available in the USA, Europe and Eire but is prohibited in the UK, other than with rats for microsurgery training. In some countries it is deemed essential that surgical experience is gained in the live, anaesthetised animal before operating on humans.[3–5]

Supervised operative experience

During any operative training a number of competing variables need to be reconciled. These variables include the skills of the trainee, which can range from beginner to well trained, the difficulty of the case selected (which is unpredictable before the laparoscope is introduced), and the time pressure to finish the operating list.

Variables competing in operative training:
- Skills of trainee
- Difficulty of selected case
- Time pressure to finish operating list

For the serious trainer this last point is the only variable that can, and *must*, be dealt with. It is dangerous to the patient, and ultimately damaging to the trainee, to be pushed through a "training procedure" because of the need to finish the list. This is an important handicap to all surgical training, but in particular to laparoscopic training. Institutions that wish to attract good surgical trainees must ensure protected operating time for training in laparoscopic surgery.

By contrast, the initial abilities of the trainee and the intra-abdominal conditions (for example, density of adhesions to the gall bladder) can not be determined by the trainer. Each apprenticeship in laparoscopic surgery is a delicate balance of supervision and demonstration until all stages of the procedure have been mastered.

Before embarking on operative apprenticeship the trainee laparoscopic surgeon should have experience in

- setting up monitors and camera;
- use of insufflator;
- handling and manipulating laparoscopic instruments;
- simulated tissue dissection and operative procedures.

The trainee should also have acted as camera operator and assistant during common laparoscopic procedures. This is an important period, in which the main stages and safety features of a procedure can be discussed with the trainee. The most common elective procedure used for teaching laparoscopic technique is laparoscopic cholecystectomy. Using this procedure as the model a number of practical stages need to be assimilated by the trainee.

Practical stages of laparoscopic cholecystectomy training:
- Insertion of Veress needle and port
- Identification and grasping of gall bladder
- Dissection of Calot's triangle
- Peroperative cholangiography
- Management of intraoperative problems

As in all surgical training, the trainer must demonstrate and then supervise each step, the safety of the patient being the first consideration. Fortunately, laparoscopic surgery is very visual and usually each decision the trainee makes can be discussed and approved by the trainer.

Management of intraoperative problems

The theoretical basis of an operative procedure can often be put across with the help of simple teaching and diagrams. If each procedure was an exact example of its kind the adage of "see one, do one, teach one" might be valid but even in laparoscopic cholecystectomy there is considerable variation in the appearance, the presence of adhesions and the difficulty of removing each gall bladder encountered. Therefore training in laparoscopic surgery is not only about how to perform the straightforward procedure but also how to manage intraoperative problems. The more cases that a trainee is exposed to under supervision the more likely he or she is to learn strategies that deal with unexpected intraoperative problems.

Potential intraoperative problems:
- Obscured anatomy
- Aberrant anatomy
- Haemorrhage

The real test of training is that the trainee can recognise an intraoperative problem and has a strategy to deal with it. In particular, the trainee should always be ready to seek intraoperative advice and/or convert the operation to an open procedure.

Videos and laparoscopic training

There are many commercial videos that allow the trainee to rehearse the steps of a laparoscopic procedure before working on a patient. It is useful to view such a video with the trainer before undertaking a laparoscopic procedure but it is even more useful to video parts of the trainee's own technique for later review. Personal records have the value of realism and the opportunity to analyse any deficiencies in technique.

How many procedures?

The number of laparoscopic procedures needed to complete the training remains the subject for debate. In laparoscopic cholecystectomy the trainee should master both the mechanics of the procedure and the approaches to the management of intraoperative problems. Such an experience might be best secured in laparoscopic cholecystectomy by the trainee acting as camera operator/assistant for ten procedures, surgeon under direct supervision for 15 procedures, and independent surgeon with the teacher in the theatre suite for a further 10 procedures. In a recent article[6] the initial experience of chief residents in the USA included 15–20 procedures as the first assistant or camera operator and a further 25–35 laporoscopic cholecystectomies as the primary surgeon. Surgeons are now completing their residency programme having performed 50–75 laparoscopic procedures as the primary surgeon. The success or otherwise of a specific training format could be established only by independent audit of a trainee's performance after leaving the trainer.

Further laparoscopic procedures

- Appendicectomy
- Hernia repair
- Nissen fundoplication

Laparoscopic cholecystectomy is the most common training operation but a series of other procedures should be learned by the trainee surgeon. These include laparoscopic appendicectomy, laparoscopic hernia repair and eventually laparoscopic Nissen fundoplication and laparoscopic colectomy. The latter two procedures are only necessary within the setting of formal specialisation in upper gastrointestinal and colorectal surgery. Training in laparoscopic appendicectomy and hernia repair can follow on from laparoscopic cholecystectomy.

Recognition and certification

A clear impetus to any formal training is recognition of that training by certification. Laparoscopic surgery is not unique among surgical techniques in requiring training, but the publicity associated with mishaps from "keyhole surgery" has caused more than usual public interest in how a surgeon acquires and uses skills. The approach from the Royal College of Surgeons of England has been to include training in laparoscopic surgery within the specialty training programmes related to the disease being treated, rather than to have a specialty training programme in "laparoscopic surgery". Thus, a surgeon would learn laparoscopic Nissen fundoplication during training (at level 2 or 3) in gastrointestinal surgery, in conjunction with other open and laparoscopic procedures on the stomach and oesophagus, and training in appropriate assessment and work-up for such patients. This should also ensure that only suitable trainees are trained in some of the more complex techniques, and that they will continue to be performed only on patients who warrant such surgery after careful assessment. The Association of Endoscopic Surgeons of Great Britain and Ireland is seeking to build a list of experienced laparoscopic surgeons who will be available to run courses for training in some of the more complex laparoscopic procedures, which should help to ensure that surgeons have adequate training before embarking on new techniques. Training at this stage would involve an experienced surgeon travelling to the trainee's hospital to train, assist and supervise the trainee's early laparoscopic experience.

Conclusions

Laparoscopic surgery offers substantial benefits to the patient over conventional surgery in several conditions. In order to make these benefits worthwhile the risks posed by laparoscopic surgery need to be minimised. This can be achieved only by realistic and comprehensive training in each technique. Protected operating time for detailed training is crucial to the laparoscopic apprenticeship in achieving this goal.

1 Royston CMS, Lansdown MRJ, Brough WA. Teaching laparoscopic surgery: the need for guidelines. *BMJ* 1994;**308**:1023–5.
2 Wolfe BM, Szabo Z, Maran ME, Chan P, Hunter JG. Training for minimally invasive surgery. Need for surgical skills. *Surg Endosc* 1993;**7**:93–5.
3 Atabek U, Spence RK, Pello MJ, Alexander JB, Villanueva D, Camishian RL. Safety of teaching laparoscopic cholecystectomy to surgical residents. *J Laparoendosc Surg* 1993;**3**:23–6.
4 Banta HD. Minimally invasive surgery. Implications for hospitals, health workers and patients. *BMJ* 1993;**307**:1546–9.
5 Clayden GS. Preliminary training on animals is essential. *BMJ* 1994;**309**:342.
6 Zucker KA, Bailey RW, Graham SM, Scovil W, Imbembo AL. Training for laparoscopic surgery. *World J Surg* 1993;**17**:3–7.

5 Use of laparoscopy in general surgery and trauma

Andrew D Clarke

Laparoscopy was used in general surgery before the laparoscopic revolution in the late 1980s. It allowed accurate diagnosis and the collection of histological material without recourse to a painful laparotomy incision. The present uses for laparoscopy in general surgery and trauma are:

- Staging of malignancy
- Ascites of unknown origin
- Liver disease
- Acute abdomen
- Trauma
- Miscellaneous

Staging of malignancy

It is important with some of the solid tumours of the gastrointestinal tract that assessment of the spread of disease is made before embarking on major surgery. Laparoscopy enables the surgeon to exclude or confirm peritoneal seedlings or hepatic spread, and allows histological confirmation of such findings. This will avoid unnecessary laparotomy in a patient with metastatic spread and also assist in optimising the use of theatre and surgeon's time. Preresection laparoscopy is particularly applicable in the management of patients with carcinoma of the stomach (Figure 5.1) or oesophagus. Ultrasound and computed tomography may lead to a false assessment of resectability, as peritoneal seedlings and small hepatic metastases can be missed. In 1984 the use of laparoscopy in such patients was reported and the surgeons were able to avoid laparotomy in 50% of patients who had been deemed suitable for surgery by other means of assessment.[1] The limitations of this assessment include the inaccessibility of the superior border of the right lobe of the liver, the difficulty of accurately assessing the posterior extension of gastric or oesophageal tumours, and the difficulty of distinguishing local tumour extension from inflammation (a problem even at laparotomy). Laparoscopy may also be used in the staging of lymphomas, to take multiple biopsies of the liver or affected lymph nodes, and to mark affected nodes with clips applied laparoscopically, thus making subsequent radiotherapy more accurate.

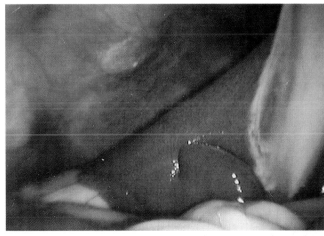
(a)

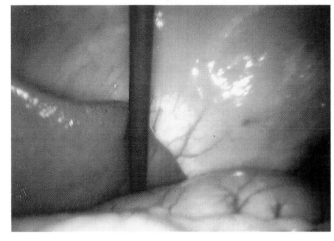
(b)

Figure 5.1 Laparoscopy for gastric carcinoma. (a) Right lobe of the liver. (b) Probe elevating left lobe of liver; the anterior aspect of the stomach is visible below this

Ascites of unknown origin

The aetiology of ascites may usually be ascertained clinically or by cytological, biochemical and microbiological assessment of the ascitic fluid. However, in about 20% of cases this is not possible. In this group laparoscopy can be used in diagnosing ascites caused by inflammatory conditions such as Crohn's disease, hepatic disease, occult intraluminal malignancy, or infections such as tuberculosis.

Liver disease[2]

Laparoscopy is the single most accurate diagnostic aid available for the hepatologist. It allows accurate assessment of hepatic nodularity, and liver biopsy can be performed under direct visualisation in order to guide the needle to the lesion requiring biopsy. This allows more accurate diagnosis, less risk of bleeding, and a therapeutic method of dealing with any bleeding that occurs by diathermy into the biopsy site. Diagnostic laparoscopy and biopsy provide the most accurate and definitive diagnosis of liver cirrhosis[3] and may depict the presence of early portal hypertension. Laparoscopy aids in the diagnosis, assessment and biopsy of primary or secondary liver tumours. In conjunction with computed tomography and ultrasound scanning the extent and spread of the disease may be seen, which is important if the patient is being considered for hepatic resection. Not uncommonly, a single metastasis seen on computed tomography is shown to be one of several deposits at laparoscopy.

The acute abdomen

The use of laparoscopy in the assessment of right iliac fossa pain is covered in Chapter 8. This is a useful tool in both male and female patients in whom diagnosis is difficult but a laparotomy is to be avoided. Laparoscopy may have a greater role in the accurate assessment of abdominal pain in children, where unclear symptomatology and vague histories can make diagnosis difficult. Laparoscopy has recently been used in the acute abdomen to diagnose conditions such as a perforated duodenal ulcer.[4] This has led to development of therapeutic manoeuvres that allow the perforation to be sutured or plugged, thus avoiding laparotomy. As more therapeutic procedures are performed laparoscopically it is likely that the laparoscope will be used more in diagnosis in the emergency situation, as some conditions seen are amenable to laparoscopic surgery.

Trauma and intensive care[2][4]

Patients who have suffered multiple trauma, or localised blunt or penetrating trauma to the abdomen may be difficult to assess initially, especially if they are unconscious. Emergency resuscitation is the priority, but accurate assessment of intraperitoneal pathology is essential for proper management. The patient may be agitated, confused, aggressive or drunk (all of which make assessment difficult), or may be unconscious or anaesthetised before a surgical assessment of the abdomen can be made. Penetrating knife or gunshot injuries can not be accurately assessed. Initial assessment

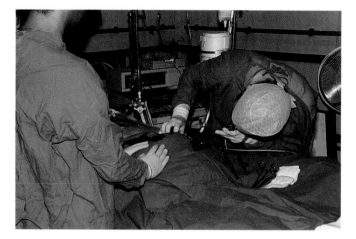

Figure 5.2 Laparoscopy in a ventilated patient in the intensive care unit

is clinical and diagnostic peritoneal lavage is often used in such patients. This shows only the level of blood in the peritoneal cavity with no indications of whether haemorrhage is continuing, which organ is bleeding or whether the bleeding needs surgical intervention. Ultrasound and computed tomography of the abdominal cavity have their use in the emergency situation, where available. Although these investigations show the presence of intraperitoneal fluid they do not differentiate between blood and other fluids such as gastrointestinal contents, and can not determine whether haemorrhage is continuing or whether the organ damage will need surgery or will resolve spontaneously. Under these circumstances laparoscopy allows accurate assessment of the amount of haemorrhage, whether it is continuing, whether it can be managed conservatively or requires resection of the damaged organ, and whether other intra-abdominal injuries such as to the gastrointestinal tract are present. In many instances this will avoid subjecting a seriously ill patient to more trauma in the shape of a laparotomy, and will enable the clinician to attend to the damaged area. Laparoscopy under local anaesthesia or sedation can be performed in emergency or intensive care departments (Figure 5.2). The use of laparoscopy reduces the negative laparotomy rate,[5] is more accurate than computed tomography and diagnostic peritoneal lavage, especially in penetrating trauma, and has additional cost saving implications.

Miscellaneous uses

A further use of laparoscopy in surgery is for the location of a testicle which is not palpable in the scrotum or groin of a child or teenager. It may be possible to locate a testicle in the retroperitoneal area, to mobilise it to allow for orchidopexy, or to remove it to prevent the increased risk of malignancy.

1 Bancewicz J *et al*. Assessment of gastric carcinoma by laparoscopy. *BMJ* 1984;**288**:1577.
2 Berci G. Elective and emergent laparoscopy. *World J Surg* 1993;**17**:8–15.
3 Orlando R, Lirussi F, Okslicsangi L, *et al*. Laparoscopy and liver biopsy—a retrospective study of 1003 consecutive examinations. *J Clin Gastroenterol* 1990;**12**:47–52.
4 Sackier JM. Laparoscopy in the emergency setting. *World J Surg* 1992;**16**:1082–8.
5 Berci G. Emergency laparoscopy. *Am J Surg* 1991;**161**:332–5.

6 Laparoscopic cholecystectomy

Timothy H Brown

Removing the gall bladder using laparoscopic techniques launched the laparoscopic revolution. In 1987 Mouret performed the first such operation[1] and this has gained widespread acceptance as the procedure of choice for removing the gall bladder. This rapid acceptance by the surgical community is probably unprecedented and has brought problems as well as benefits. In this chapter we shall deal with the technique for performing a laparoscopic cholecystectomy (LC), including the approach to difficult cases, and the complications that may arise.

Patient selection

It is important that the same selection criteria apply to LC as to open cholecystectomy: the patient must have symptomatic gall stones or gall bladder disease. It is not enough to demonstrate the presence of gall stones, as a number of patients with these have no problems ("silent" gall stones). In the USA the total cost of surgery for gall bladder disease has risen since the introduction of LC, despite the fact that it is cheaper than open cholecystectomy. This is because the number of procedures being performed is increasing, and we must protect against this increase or we risk a good operation acquiring a bad reputation due to operating unnecessarily, poor laparoscopic technique, or a complication arising following an unnecessary procedure.

A careful history and examination of the patient should be undertaken, followed by ultrasound scanning of the gall bladder, and liver function tests. If the scan confirms gall stones, if the blood tests are normal, and if the symptoms fit with the diagnosis of biliary disease, then the possibility of LC should be discussed with the patient. This should include an explanation of the procedure, its benefits, and its risks. If the ultrasound scan shows a dilated common bile duct or suggests stones in the duct, or if the liver function tests suggest some degree of obstructive jaundice, the initial approach should be endoscopic retrograde cholangiopancreatography (ERCP), with sphincterotomy and stone extraction if required. Caution should be exercised with young patients requiring a sphincterotomy because of the risks of the procedure (pancreatitis, haemorrhage, duodenal leak) and the possible long term sequelae. Once the need for LC is confirmed, the patient should be submitted for surgery. In certain conditions LC is more difficult to perform; these will be discussed at the appropriate place in the text.

Operative technique

A LC is performed under general anaesthesia with the patient supine on the operating table. The operating room is set up as shown in Figure 6.1, with the surgeon standing on the patient's left, the camera operator to the surgeon's left and a second assistant (if used) opposite the surgeon alongside the scrub nurse. The main monitor is placed to the right of the patient's head (Figure 6.2), and a second (optional) monitor to their left. The insufflator, light source and camera attachments may be placed under the main monitor, thus keeping the room tidy. The suction/irrigator is held in a quiver near the patient's head (Figure 6.3) with the giving set and suction tubing passing out together to the irrigation fluid and suction apparatus respectively. One litre of irrigation fluid should contain 10 000 units of heparin and a suitable antibiotic (1 g tetracycline). The tubing (light lead, camera cable, gas supply) should be held securely, to keep them away from the area of surgery and maintain sterility.

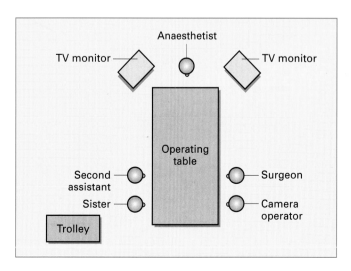

Figure 6.1 Plan of the operating room set up for laparoscopic cholecystectomy

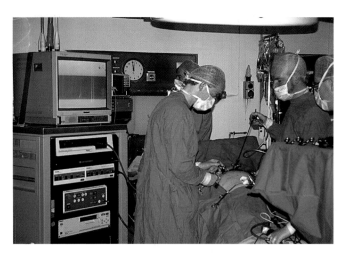

Figure 6.2 Surgeon, assistants and equipment for laparoscopic cholecystectomy

Pneumoperitoneum and port placement

The initial 1 cm incision is made at the umbilicus, transversely or longitudinally. In order to assist with introducing the Veress needle and the umbilical port sutures may be placed on the anterior rectus sheath. This sheath is grasped and retracted upwards with Allis forceps (Figure 6.4) and sutures are placed each side of the midline. These are used to elevate the anterior abdominal wall (Figure 6.3) while introducing the Veress needle and the 10 mm port and may be ligated at the end of the procedure to close the midline defect. The Veress needle is introduced carefully, ensuring that two layers are passed through with the minimum risk of damage to underlying structures. A syringe containing saline solution is used to check for correct placement, and carbon dioxide (CO_2) introduced at 1 l/min. Once the CO_2 flow is satisfactory and the intra-abdominal pressure remains low (below 10 mmHg), the flow may be raised to 4 l/min until the peritoneal cavity is suitably distended (usually 3–4 litres is needed). The Veress needle is then withdrawn and a 10 mm port introduced, to which the gas insufflation tubing is attached. The laparoscope is introduced and the peritoneal cavity

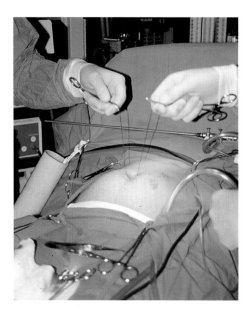

Figure 6.3 Sutures placed for elevation—also note quiver for instruments

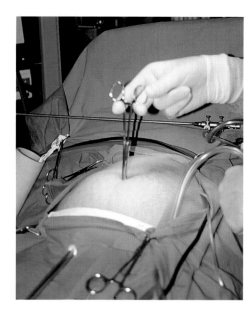

Figure 6.4 Allis forceps placed on the midline

inspected, to assess whether the laparoscopic procedure is possible and to look for other disease. The fundus of the gall bladder may be visible at this stage (Figure 6.5). The other three ports are placed under direct vision: a 10 mm port is placed in the epigastrium and directed through the falciform ligament towards the right side of the abdomen, a 5 mm port is placed midway along the costal margin on the right (slightly below the ribs), and the fourth port (5 mm) is introduced in the anterior axillary line also just below the ribs.

Instruments and their position

The laparoscope is introduced via the umbilical port. The CO_2 may be passed via this port, although, if it causes excessive misting of the lens, it may be moved to another port. The epigastric port is the main operating port and is used for the grasping forceps, the scissors, the diathermy hook, the suction/irrigator, and the clip applier, most of which are introduced via a reducing port. The third (5 mm) port is used for a pair of ratcheted grasping forceps to hold the gall bladder at Hartmann's pouch and to retract it laterally and anteriorly. Forceps are introduced via the fourth port to

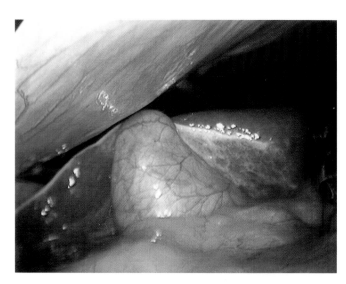

Figure 6.5 Fundus of the gall bladder visible in the right upper quadrant, just beneath the liver

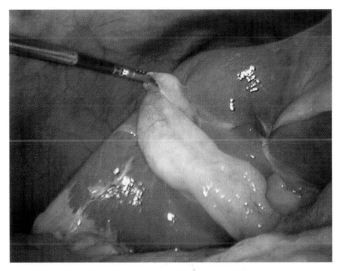

Figure 6.6 Fundus of the gall bladder grasped and pushed over the liver edge

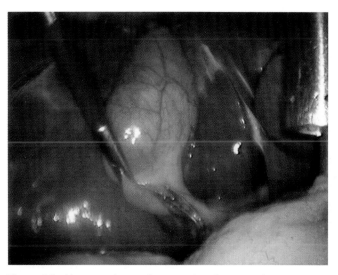

Figure 6.7 Hartmann's pouch grasped and retracted

grasp the fundus of the gall bladder and distract it towards the right shoulder, over the superior border of the liver (Figure 6.6). This procedure may be very difficult if the gall bladder is grossly enlarged or its wall is thick. An empyema or mucocoele may cause this, and accompanying inflammation and adhesions will add to the problem. Aspiration of the fluid contents of the gall bladder will often make grasping the fundus easier, and it is usually best to place the forceps over the hole made by the aspirating needle. The surgeon should remember that a gall bladder that has been aspirated should be extracted using a retrieval bag (see below).

The operating table is adjusted to bring the gall bladder into vision by elevating the head end of the table and raising the right side. This allows the stomach and small intestine to fall to the left or to the lower peritoneal cavity and brings the gall bladder into the centre of the picture.

Obtaining good gall bladder position

Dissecting forceps are introduced via the epigastric port to assist forceps passed via the fourth port in grasping the fundus. The fundus is pushed up over the anterior border of the liver (Figure 6.6) and adhesions between the gall bladder and the omentum, bowel or mesentery are stripped away, diathermied or divided to allow further retraction of the fundus. As Hartmann's pouch becomes visible it should be grasped by a second instrument and retracted to stretch Calot's triangle (Figure 6.7). A little irrigation fluid introduced at this stage will ensure that any blood spilt remains unclotted, and thus easier to aspirate. The box lists some laparoscopic findings that can make LC more difficult.

- Adhesions—umbilical, intraperitoneal, perihepatic, or to the gall bladder
- Enlarged gall bladder; for example, empyema or mucocoele
- Stone impacted in Hartmann's pouch
- Inflammation in Calot's triangle
- Stones in the common bile duct or common hepatic duct
- Aberrant anatomy
- Stone spillage

Intraperitoneal adhesions

Intraperitoneal adhesions in the upper half of the abdomen can make peritoneal insufflation, visualisation, mobilisation, and surgery of the gall bladder very difficult. These adhesions are usually secondary to previous surgery or inflammation and cause problems with peritoneal insufflation.

Insufflation

Adhesions to the umbilicus can lead to an elevation of the inflation pressure when insufflation is attempted, alerting the surgeon to this possibility. The problem can usually be overcome by repositioning the needle in the right or left upper quadrants, although blind attempts may risk damage to underlying bowel. Should this fail, the wound at the umbilicus should be opened under direct vision (Hassan approach), the peritoneum visualised and incised, the port introduced without its trocar, and held in place using a purse string suture.

Right upper quadrant adhesions

Adhesions in the right upper quadrant due to small intestine or colon held to the anterior abdominal wall may obscure visualisation of the gall bladder. These may be divided at their attachment to the anterior abdominal wall using scissors, hook diathermy or laser, but if this is not possible the laparoscope may be passed through a non-vascular window in these adhesions and the other ports placed under direct vision. If an adequate laparoscopic view of the gall bladder can not be obtained open operation is more appropriate.

Perihepatic adhesions

Adhesions to the liver or gall bladder are fairly common and can usually be divided, diathermied or stripped away, using diathermy to control bleeding. In some cases of empyema of the gall bladder, or severe inflammation, the adhesions can not be freed laparoscopically. If a plane is found between the adhesions and the gall bladder a hook diathermy can be inserted and the plane extended along the length of the gall bladder, keeping close to the gall bladder rather than the adhesions (inadvertently producing a hole in the gall bladder is better than damaging the bowel). This is especially true in the region of the duodenum, and in Calot's triangle, where the ductal structures may be hidden in the adhesions.

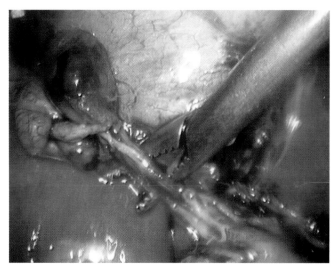

Figure 6.8 Dissecting forceps opened to separate tissue in Calot's triangle

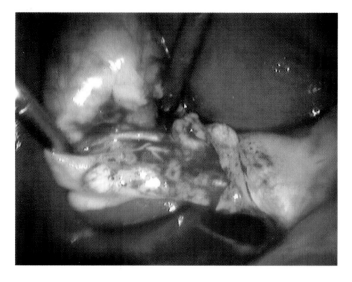

(a)

Calot's triangle

This is the most important part of the dissection and it is imperative that the anatomy here is clearly defined before anything is divided. Adhesions, bleeding, poor retraction, inflammation, or a distended gall bladder increase the difficulty of determining the anatomy and if a clear view is not possible the procedure should be converted to an open procedure before any permanent damage is inflicted. As with an open procedure, it is important to define the cystic duct and cystic artery and to ensure that the common bile duct and common hepatic duct are away from the operative field. Calot's triangle is cleared, using grasping forceps to strip tissue from the gall bladder, by dividing the peritoneum over Hartmann's pouch using hook diathermy, or by using pressure irrigation to separate the tissues. The dissecting forceps are opened to help define the duct and artery (Figure 6.8) and as the cystic duct becomes visible it is traced to its attachment to the gall bladder, noting where it widens at the gall bladder neck. It may be possible to see the cystic duct and common bile duct junction, but this is not usually the case. The cystic artery should also be identified and cleared, but it is not always possible to do this before the cystic duct is divided. The tissue between the liver bed and the gall bladder can be separated to help outline the cystic duct and artery as they pass to the gall bladder. This helps to clarify whether the duct identified is single or a loop. Inflammation and adhesions in Calot's triangle can be a real challenge: the surgeon must not continue if the anatomy is unclear, but what may seem initially to be impossible (Figure 6.9a) may become clear after careful dissection (Figure 6.9b and c). Dissection between the gall bladder and liver bed at this stage may improve visibility, as may approaching Calot's triangle from beneath the gall bladder.

If a large stone is impacted in Hartmann's pouch distorted anatomy may make clearing Calot's triangle difficult. Under these circumstances dissection should proceed close to the gall bladder wall, peeling adhesions and inflamed tissue away until the ductal structures are visible at their junction with the gall bladder.

Peroperative cholangiography

Once the cystic duct has been identified a clip should be placed at its junction with the gall bladder (Figure

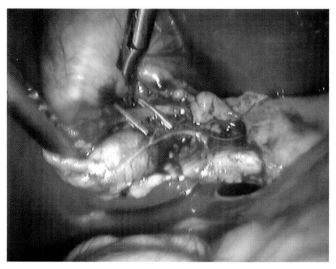

(b)

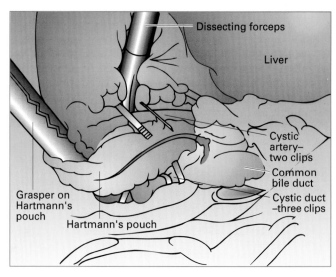

(c)

Figure 6.9 (a) Calot's triangle during early dissection. Note that the anatomy is not clear. (b) and (c) Calot's triangle after careful dissection. The cystic artery and cystic duct are now seen more clearly and have been clipped

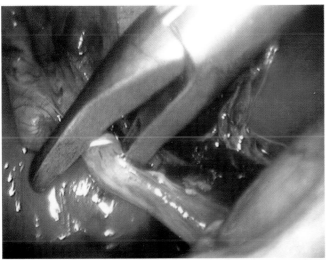

Figure 6.10 Clip being placed on the cystic duct near the gall bladder

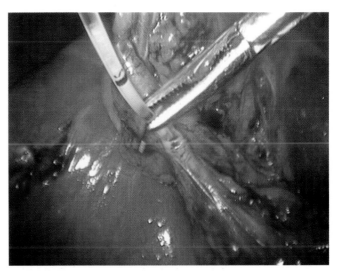

(a)

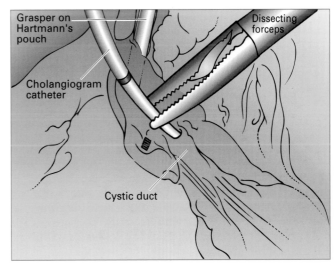

(b)

Figure 6.12 Cholangiogram catheter in the cystic duct

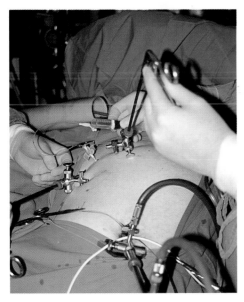

Figure 6.11 Umbilical catheter placed via Venflon for cholangiogram

6.10) and a small cut made just proximal to the clip through which a cholangiogram catheter is introduced. The simplest technique is to place a 14 G Venflon (BOC Ohmeda AB, Sweden) through the anterior abdominal wall between the third and fourth ports, and to introduce a size 4 umbilical catheter preloaded with radio-opaque dye (Figure 6.11). The catheter is grasped and guided into the cystic duct (Figure 6.12); holding the catheter in place by a clip across the duct will prevent its dislodgement but will still allow flow of contrast into the biliary system. The instruments are removed and cholangiograms obtained using 5 and 10 ml of contrast to demonstrate the anatomy (Figure 6.13), to show flow into the hepatic radicles, filling of the common bile duct, dye in the duodenum, and the presence of any stones. If concerned about the anatomy, bile duct damage, or stones the surgeon must decide whether to proceed or to use open surgery. Once the radiograph has been taken the clip and the cholangiogram catheter are removed.

Stones in the biliary system

- Explore duct laparoscopically
- Perform ERCP and stone extraction in theatre
- Finish laparoscopic cholecystectomy, postoperative ERCP
- Convert to open exploration of common bile duct

These can be managed in a number of different ways. If the surgeon has a wide experience of laparoscopic procedures then laparoscopic exploration of the common bile duct may be attempted[23] using the cystic duct as the means of entry.[4] This duct is dilated to enable introduction of a flexible choledochoscope or ureteroscope. The stones are removed using a Dormia basket, pushed into the duodenum or fragmented using a lithotripter. The common bile duct may also be explored laparoscopically by incising it longitudinally, much as would be done at open operation. Should these techniques not be possible or advisable then the stones may be removed via an ERCP and sphincterotomy either in theatre (though this usually creates logistic difficulties),

23

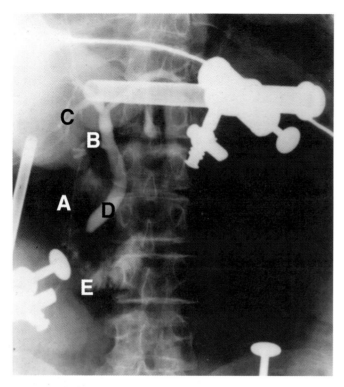

Figure 6.13 Peroperative cholangiogram. A, catheter; B, cystic duct; C, intrahepatic ducts; D, common bile duct; E, dye in the duodenum

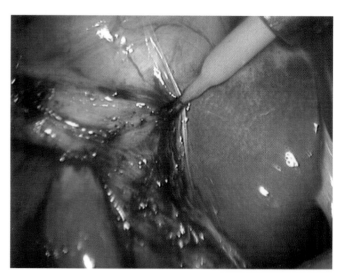

Figure 6.15 Gall bladder (pushed up to the patient's right) being separated from the liver using diathermy hook

or postoperatively. The disadvantage with the postoperative approach is that it may prove impossible to extract the stones via ERCP, and so a second surgical procedure will be required. If these approaches are deemed unsuitable, the LC should be converted to an open operation and the duct explored further.

Dividing the cystic duct and artery

Two clips should be placed on the proximal cystic duct and the duct divided between these and the clip near the gall bladder (Figure 6.14). Scissors should be used rather than diathermy as the current may be conducted along the cystic duct and clips and cause thermal damage to the cystic or common bile duct. The

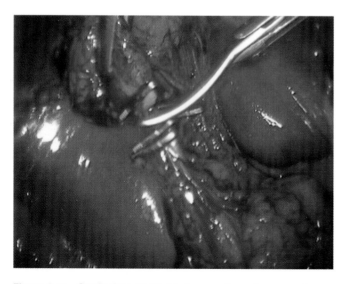

Figure 6.14 Cystic duct divided between clips using curved scissors

cystic artery is clipped and divided, leaving one or two clips. The gall bladder may now be retracted away from the liver.

Aberrant anatomy

Anatomical textbooks show the variety of anatomy of Calot's triangle and the interrelationships of the gall bladder, cystic duct, common hepatic duct, common bile duct, cystic artery, and right hepatic artery. It is imperative that the surgeon appreciates these variations and that at LC the ducts and vessels are clearly identified, including any aberrant ducts or vessels. No tubular structure should be clipped until the surgeon is certain what it is, where it is going and what its relationships are to surrounding structures. The cystic duct should be identified by its junction with the gall bladder. It is sometimes possible to identify the junction of the cystic duct with the common bile duct, but it is inadvisable to dissect in this area if the anatomy is not clear, as damage to the common bile duct or its vascular supply may occur. If, during LC, the surgeon can not properly identify the anatomy he or she should seek senior help, or convert to an open cholecystectomy.

Removal of the gall bladder

The gall bladder is separated from the liver bed using a hook diathermy (Figure 6.15), scissors, laser,[5] or pressurised irrigation. Attempts should be made to avoid holing the gall bladder and spilling bile or stones, and dissection into the liver (which can cause excessive bleeding) should also be avoided. Spilt bile can be irrigated and aspirated. Spillage of stones is common during LC as the gall bladder may be torn or split while it is being grasped at the fundus or Hartmann's pouch, while it is being dissected from the liver bed, or during its extraction. A recent report[6] suggests that this can occur in up to one third of patients undergoing LC.

Dealing with spilled stones

The approach to dealing with stone spillage varies: a small tear may be controlled by grasping the hole with a pair of forceps, or by closing the defect with an Endoloop (Ethicon Endosurgery, Edinburgh, UK);[7] a larger tear can be controlled by placing Endoloops on each side to close the defect and prevent spillage.

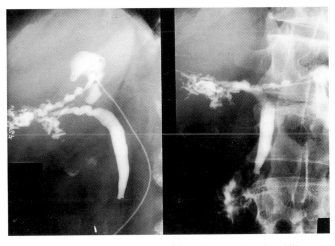

Figure 6.16 Fistulogram from epigastric port, showing biliary connection

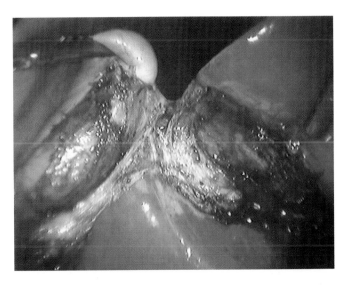

Figure 6.17 The gall bladder has been retracted to demonstrate the liver bed

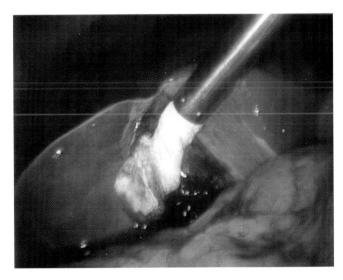

Figure 6.18 Haemostatic material placed in the liver bed

Should a tear occur the gall bladder should be extracted in a retrieval bag, such as a "Bert" bag (Vernon Carus, Preston, UK), to avoid further tearing and stone spillage during extraction. Retrieval of a few spilled stones should be attempted using grasping forceps or a Dormia basket,[8] through a reducing port. If several stones are spilled then a retrieval bag should be introduced into the peritoneum and the stones placed in the bag before being removed. This may be tedious but is possible with increasing skill. Many tiny stones may be irrigated with saline and aspirated via the suction/irrigation device. Some surgeons leave the stones in the peritoneal cavity but complications arising from these include intraperitoneal abscess,[8] biliary fistulation,[9] and trocar site abscess.[10] Figure 6.16 shows a fistulous connection from the epigastric port to the biliary tree resulting from retained stone fragments in the peritoneal cavity coupled with the presence of bile from the cystic duct. On balance, spilled stones should be retrieved, especially if they are fragmented, but it may be safe to leave multiple small stones. If there is any concern about leaving stones then the laparoscopic procedure should be converted to an open procedure.

Before dividing the final attachment of the gall bladder to the liver bed, the gall bladder may be used as a retractor to elevate the liver so that the gall bladder bed can be irrigated and checked for haemorrhage (Figure 6.17). Any haemorrhage from the liver bed may be stopped by diathermy, pressure (using a pledget), or by placing haemostatic material (such as Oxycel, or Surgicel) into the liver bed via a 10 mm port (Figure 6.18).

Extraction of the gall bladder

The gall bladder is extracted most easily via the epigastric port using a large pair of grasping forceps (Figure 6.19). Some surgeons prefer to use the umbilical port, as it can be widened leaving a less obvious scar, but this requires the laparoscope to be moved from the umbilical to the epigastric port and the surgeon to reorient the direction and angles of the instruments. If the gall bladder has been holed, is very friable, or will be difficult to remove then it should be placed in a "Bert" bag before removal (Figure 6.20). Manipulation of the gall bladder into this bag can be difficult, but a greater degree of traction can be put on the "Bert" bag than on the gall bladder and once at the skin the bag can be opened and bile aspirated, stones extracted, or the gall bladder removed piecemeal. The port can be enlarged using dilators or by dividing rectus sheath or skin.

After the gall bladder has been extracted the port is replaced, the operation site rechecked and irrigated and the irrigation fluid and blood aspirated. If there is

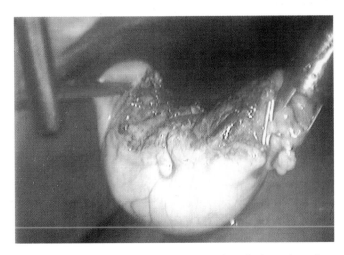

Figure 6.19 Gall bladder ready for extraction via the epigastric port

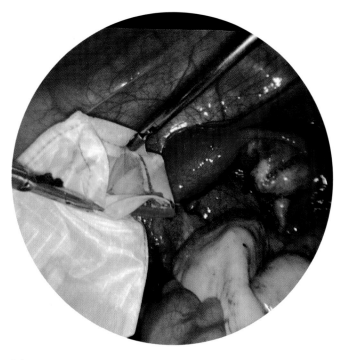

(a)

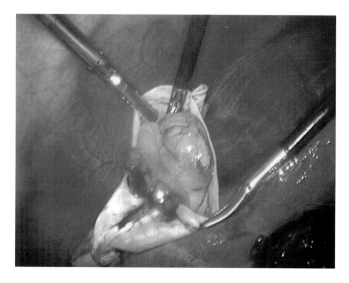

(b)

Figure 6.20 (a) "Bert" bag opened in the peritoneal cavity. (b) Gall bladder placed in "Bert" bag

continued oozing, or contamination with bile or pus, a drain should be introduced via the fourth port and positioned using the grasping forceps.

Closure

The two 5 mm ports and the epigastric port are removed under direct vision and the CO_2 allowed to escape from the peritoneal cavity. The umbilical port is removed and the sutures that had been placed earlier held up to allow any remaining CO_2 to escape. These two sutures are ligated to close the umbilical defect, and sutures are placed in the rectus sheath to close the epigastric port. The wounds are then irrigated with antibiotic irrigation fluid and the skin closed with sutures or clips.

Complications

- Haemorrhage
- Bile leakage (abscess, collection, fistula)
- Bile duct injury
- Vascular and visceral injuries
- Retained intraductal stones
- Retained intraperitoneal stones
- Wound hernia
- Tumour implantation

Haemorrhage

The extent of haemorrhage occuring during laparoscopic surgery may be difficult to assess for two reasons: firstly, the magnification on the monitor tends to exaggerate the degree of haemorrhage, and secondly, the blood absorbs light, thus reducing illumination and visibility. Haemorrhage is controlled using diathermy, clips, Endoloops or pressure. Oozing from the liver bed is usually stopped by diathermy but other techniques may be required, including pressure with a pledget or the placement of haemostatic material via a reducing port (Figure 6.18), which aids haemostasis and may be left in the abdomen at the end of the procedure. A suction drain can be inserted via the right flank port to enable aspiration of residual fluid; fluid left here may become infected and lead to a subphrenic abscess.

Bile leakage

Bile can leak from the cystic duct stump, a hole in the common bile or common hepatic duct, a bile radicle in the liver bed, or an aberrant bile duct inadvertently divided. As a result bile may leak through the drain or form a biloma, an abscess (if infected) or a biliary fistula may develop. Bile duct injury is more common after LC than after open cholecystectomy. If bile leakage occurs the drain should be left in place until the bile drainage ceases, usually within a day or two. Further investigation is required if the drainage persists.

Bile in the peritoneal cavity may form a collection (biloma) or distribute through the peritoneal cavity (bile ascites or biliary peritonitis).[11] Bile leakage into the peritoneum occurs if the clip dislodges from the cystic duct stump, if a hole has been made in the cystic duct proximal to the clip, in the common hepatic or common bile duct, or an aberrant duct from the liver to the cystic duct has been divided. The patient may still be an inpatient when leakage occurs, or may return complaining of right upper quadrant pain, malaise or lethargy. Investigation, by ultrasonography or computed tomographic scanning, will identify any fluid collection suitable for aspiration under ultrasound guidance and a drain should be placed until the leakage dries up. Should drainage persist or recur, an ERCP may show leakage from the cystic duct stump (Figure 6.21), or the bile ducts. Treatment is by sphincterotomy or stent placement, especially if there is evidence of hold up to bile flow at the distal end of the common bile duct. Occasionally, a laparotomy may be needed to stop a persistent bile leak.

In a patient presenting with persistent pain and a swinging temperature an infection in a collection of bile may have caused a subphrenic abscess. Investigation and treatment is similar to that required for treating a non-infected biloma.

A persistent bile leak, usually with an obstructed bile duct or in the presence of an intra-abdominal nidus of infection, may lead to fistulation from a port site (Figure 6.16). Treatment is by ERCP and stenting, or by repair at open operation.

Bile duct injury

Bile duct injury is a serious complication which occurs more commonly after LC than after open cholecystectomy.[12] Investigations include ultrasonography (to diagnose a fluid collection and aspirate it if appropriate), scintigraphy (to determine a persistent biliary leak), and ERCP (to identify and treat the injury).[13 14] Damage may include a side hole in the common bile or hepatic duct caused by dissection or diathermy close to the duct. Conducted current may directly damage the duct or damage the vascular supply and lead to wall ischaemia.[15]

A bile duct stricture (Figure 6.22) may occur if a clip partially occludes or erodes into the duct.[16] This can occur if clips are placed blindly in an attempt to control haemorrhage in Calot's triangle (an unwise manoeuvre), or if the common bile duct is clipped instead of the cystic duct. The stricture is often not detected during the procedure and the patient develops epigastric or right upper quadrant pain, obstructive jaundice, or ascending cholangitis. Investigation is by ultrasonography and ERCP, and the stricture managed with an endoscopically placed stent (Figure 6.23). If the problem is noticed during the operation the patient should be opened, the clips removed and the cholecystectomy completed. Even so, a stricture may result from ischaemic damage, so long term follow up is required.

Division of the bile duct

The incidence of bile duct division during LC is just under 1% in large series,[17 18] 4–10 times more common than at open operation. It occurs when the common bile duct is mistaken for the cystic duct (gall bladder distraction causing distortion of the anatomy), clipped and divided. If this mistake is realised at the time of operation the procedure is converted to an open

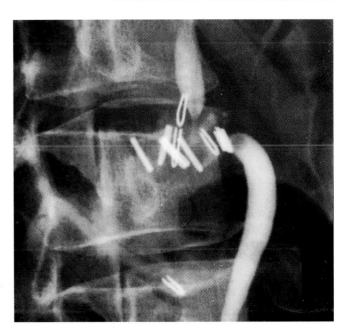

Figure 6.22 Bile duct stricture in the region of clips

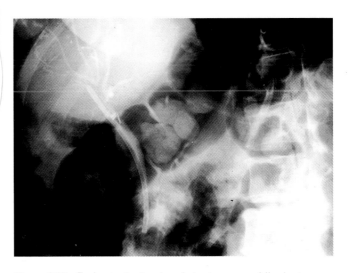

Figure 6.23 Endoscopically placed stent across a bile duct stricture

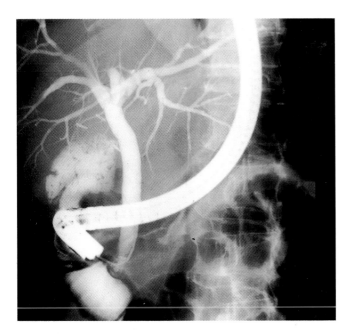

Figure 6.21 ERCP showing leak from the junction of the cystic duct and the common bile duct

procedure to perform primary repair or end-to-side hepaticodochojejunostomy. Even if immediate repair is performed a stricture may still result (Figure 6.24). Delayed presentation can include jaundice or signs of a right upper quadrant collection (pain and a temperature). Assessment by ultrasonography and ERCP (Figure 6.25) will confirm the diagnosis. The patient should be transferred to the care of a surgeon who specialises in reconstructive biliary surgery.

Vascular/visceral injuries

These injuries are rare, vascular injuries occurring in 0·25% and bowel injuries in 0·14% in a large series.[18] The former usually follow a puncture injury at insertion of the Veress needle or trocar, but bleeding can also be due to excessive retraction or adhesiolysis. Injuries to the small bowel or colon may occur during the introduction of the Veress needle or trocars, or result from retraction. Diathermy may cause a thermal injury due to direct contact or conduction,[19] which may present as a delayed perforation with septic complications.

These injuries are among the most serious after laparoscopic surgery; in one series 18 of 33 deaths

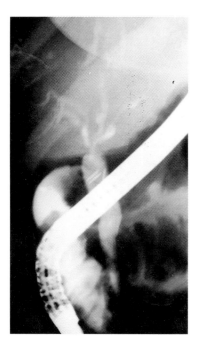

Figure 6.24 Long term stricture following division and early repair of the common bile duct

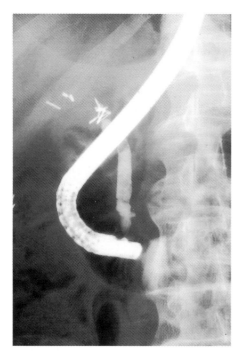

Figure 6.25 ERCP showing occlusion of the common bile duct with a clip

following LC were due to operative injury,[18] of which seven were due to haemorrhage (aorta, gall bladder bed, hepatic artery, portal vein) and five to bowel injury (colon, small bowel, duodenum) with mortality rates of 3·6% and 4·6% respectively.

Retained intraductal stone

Patients present with pain in the right upper quadrant (often similar to that experienced before surgery), obstructive jaundice, or ascending cholangitis. Ultrasonography and ERCP usually give an accurate diagnosis, and stones may be extracted at ERCP after sphincterotomy. If this is unsuccessful open exploration of the common bile duct is necessary.

Retained intraperitoneal stones

Most spilled stones remain asymptomatic but occasionally complications arise. These include intraperitoneal abscess,[20] discharge of the stone via a cannula site,[21] or a cutaneous–biliary fistula. Treatment involves ultrasound guided drainage or open operation and drainage.

Wound herniation

The incidence of herniation through the entry wounds would be expected to be low, but failure to close the defect at the umbilical wound has led to herniation and small bowel obstruction. This complication may be minimised by closing these wounds after operation.

Tumour implantation

There have been reports of malignant cell implantation at trocar sites following laparoscopic surgery,[22] due to a carcinoma of the gall bladder or biliary system or to an unknown intraperitoneal malignancy. Malignant tissue should be extracted in an impervious bag to prevent wound implantation but it is difficult to protect completely against implantation. if the history of a patient undergoing LC suggests malignancy then a thorough inspection of the peritoneal cavity should be undertaken before proceeding, and the presence of malignant disease necessitates an open operation.

1 Mouret G. From the first laparoscopic cholecystectomy to the frontiers of laparoscopic surgery: the future perspective. *Dig Surg* 1991;**8**:124–5.
2 Petelin JB. Laparoscopic approach to common duct pathology. *Surg Laparosc Endosc* 1991;**1**:33–41.
3 Martin IG, Curley P, McMahon MJ. Minimally invasive treatment for common bile duct stones. *Br J Surg* 1993;**80**:103–6.
4 Bagnato VJ. Laparoscopic choledochoscopy and choledocholithotomy. *Surg Laparosc Endosc* 1993;**3**:164–6.
5 Spaer AT, Reddick EJ, Olsen DO. Laparoscopic laser cholecystectomy: analysis of 500 procedures. *Surg Laparosc Endosc* 1991;**1**:27.
6 Soper NJ, Dunnegan DL. Does intraoperative gall bladder perforation influence the early outcome of laparoscopic cholecystectomy. *Surg Laparosc Endosc* 1991;**1**:156–61.
7 Welch NT, Hinder RA, Ciuris T, Bacon N. Laparoscopic capture of "escaped" gallstones. *Surg Laparosc Endosc* 1991;**1**:42–4.
8 Leslie KA, Rankin RN, Duff JH. Lost gallstones during laparoscopic cholecystectomy: are they really benign? *Can J Surg* 1994;**37**:240–2.
9 Issac J, Tekant Y, Kum CK, Ngoi SS, Goh P. Endoscopic sphincterotomy for the treatment of cystic duct leak following laparoscopic cholecystectomy. *Surg Laparosc Endosc* 1994;**4**:125–7.
10 Dreznik Z, Soper NJ. Trocar site abscess due to spilled gallstones: an unusual late complication of laparoscopic cholecystectomy. *Surg Laparosc Endosc* 1993;**3**:223–4.
11 Howell DA, Bosco JJ, Sampson LN, Bula V. Endoscopic management of cystic duct fistulas after laparoscopic cholecystectomy. *Endoscopy* 1992;**24**:796–8.
12 Macintyre IMC, Wilson RG. Laparoscopic cholecystectomy. *Br J Surg* 1993;**80**:552–9.
13 Windsor JA, Vokes DE. Early laparoscopic biliary injury: experience in New Zealand. *Br J Surg* 1994;**81**:1208–11.
14 Vitale GC, Stephens G, Wieman TJ, Larson GM. Use of endoscopic retrograde cholangiopancreaticogram in the management of biliary complications after laparoscopic cholecystectomy. *Surgery* 1993;**114**:806–14.
15 O'Hanlon DM, O'Donoghue JM, Flynn JR. Unusual biliary injury following laparoscopic cholecystectomy. *Br J Surg* 1994;**81**:136–7.
16 Birks E, Tate JJT, Dooley JS, Davidson BR. Occult biliary injury after laparoscopic cholecystectomy. *Br J Surg* 1994;**81**:1366–7.
17 Go PMNYH, Schol F, Gouma DJ. Laparoscopic cholecystectomy in the Netherlands. *Br J Surg* 1993;**80**:1180–3.
18 Deziel DJ, Millikan KW, Economou SG, Doolas A, Ko S-T, Airan MC. Complications of laparoscopic cholecystectomy: a national survey of 4292 hospitals and an analysis of 77 604 cases. *Am J Surg* 1993;**165**:9–14.
19 Berry SM, Ose KJ, Bell RH, Fink AS. Thermal injury of the posterior duodenum during laparoscopic cholecystectomy. *Surg Endosc* 1994;**8**:197–200.
20 Catarci M, Zaraca F, Scaccia M, Carboni M. Lost intraperitoneal stones after laparoscopic cholecystectomy: harmless sequela or reason for reoperation. *Surg Laparosc Endosc* 1993;**3**:318–22.
21 Guy PR, Watkin DS, Thompson MH. Late discharge of stones after laparoscopic cholecystectomy. *Br J Surg* 1993;**80**:1052.
22 Pezet D, Fondrinier E, Rotman N, Guy L, Lemesle P, Lointier P, Chipponi J. Parietal seeding of carcinoma of the gall bladder after laparoscopic cholecystectomy. *Br J Surg* 1992;**79**:230.

7 Laparoscopic repair of groin hernias

J Hill, R C Pearson, I MacLennan

Annually 80 000 groin hernias are repaired and 40 000 trusses are prescribed in the UK.[1] The surgical techniques used are varied, as are the recurrence rates (<1% to >20%),[2–7] but the aim of these procedures is to prevent the herniation of intra-abdominal contents into the groin or the scrotum.

- Bassini repair—"conventional"
- Shouldice technique
- Lichtenstein repair—low tension, prosthetic
- Laparoscopic mesh repair

The defect leading to the herniation is either anatomical, with a persistence of the path from the descent of the testicle, or physiological, with a weakness in the musculature of the posterior wall of the inguinal canal.

The surgical aims are twofold:

- to ligate any sac that has developed;
- to strengthen the posterior wall of the inguinal canal.

The second aim can be achieved by plicating the conjoint tendon down towards the inguinal ligament to close the posterior wall defect, and to hold this in place using non-absorbable suture (Bassini repair). The disadvantage of this is that the anatomical defect is corrected only by using a degree of tension. A second approach repairs the posterior wall defect by using the strong fascial layer (Shouldice repair). This technique involves less tissue tension and has a lower recurrence rate in experienced hands[3] but is more complicated to learn. A third technique, now widely employed, is the use of a low tension prosthetic mesh repair (Lichtenstein repair).[5 6] Using this approach a prosthetic mesh is placed over the defect in the posterior wall of the inguinal canal and held in place with a combination of interrupted and continuous non-absorbable sutures. Laparoscopic hernia repair similarly uses a prosthetic mesh repair over the defect, thus obtaining a tension free repair, but the approach is via the peritoneal cavity and addresses the anatomical defect directly rather than disturbing the skin, subcutaneous fat, fascia and musculoaponeurotic layer of the inguinal canal.

The principles of who should undergo hernia repair and which technique should be used are discussed in guidelines issued by the Royal College of Surgeons of England.[1] The various techniques possible are described in a number of textbooks and articles, especially a recent publication by Arregui and Nagan.[8]

Advantages and disadvantages

The potential advantages of laparoscopic herniorrhaphy are not as obvious as those of laparoscopic cholecystectomy.

- Attacks area of inherent weakness
- Leaves cord structures in place
- Useful in recurrence after conventional repair
- Early mobilisation and return to work

Anatomy

A synthetic mesh is inserted between the peritoneum and the transversalis fascia (the anatomical site of the defect), directly addressing the inherent weakness without disturbing the superficial layers or the cord structures.

Anaesthesia

Conventional hernia repair is performed under general, regional, or local anaesthesia; laparoscopic repair requires general, or possibly epidural, anaesthesia. Surgeons are encouraged to perform up to 30% of open repairs as day cases,[9] and laparoscopic repair can also be performed as a day case procedure.

Recovery

After open repair patients may return to work and normal activity within 2 weeks, but usually take much longer. Laparoscopic repair avoids a groin incision, reducing postoperative pain and allowing an accelerated return to work. The patient usually returns to work about 1 week after laparoscopic repair.[10–12]

Recurrence

Recurrence after open repair is 1–20%. Of the 10 000 hernias repaired in the UK private sector 10% are performed for recurrence; this is a generally agreed global recurrence rate for conventional repairs, most of which occur within 2 years of primary surgery. Experience with laparoscopic repair suggests recurrence rates of about 1% in the first 2 years.[10–13] Wide achievement of this rate would give laparoscopic techniques a strong advantage over conventional techniques.

Technique

A variety of techniques have been attempted. Initially, plugs of synthetic material were pushed into the hernial defect and inguinal canal but this technique has been abandoned because it caused pain, migration, and early recurrence.[14] The defect should be covered with a synthetic, non-absorbable mesh (such as Prolene), which is most easily applied by suturing or stapling in position directly over the defect without peritoneal cover.[15 16] However, leaving a mesh without peritoneal cover is associated with the risk of bowel or bladder adherence to the mesh and subsequent fistulation.

Transabdominal preperitoneal repair (TAPP)

This technique is the most widely accepted laparoscopic repair. It is performed under general anaesthesia with muscle relaxation. A prophylactic dose of antibiotic should be administered at induction of anaesthesia.[13] The patient's bladder should be emptied before commencement.

Set up and positioning

A Veress needle is inserted just below the umbilicus to obtain a pneumoperitoneum with an intra-abdominal pressure of 10 mmHg. The surgeon stands opposite the hernia with the monitor on the hernial side across the operating field to allow hand and eye coordination in the same direction. The assistant holding the laparoscope stands caudal or opposite to the surgeon, who performs the procedure with both hands. Figure 7.1 shows the positions of theatre staff for performing a left inguinal

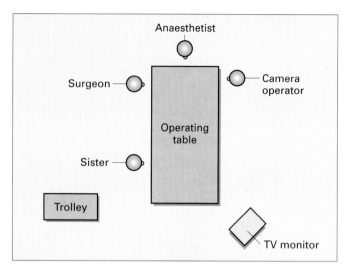

Figure 7.2 Plan of theatre set up for left inguinal hernia repair

hernia repair. The surgeon is on the right of the picture, just to the right of the patient's head. Figure 7.2 shows a plan of the set up.

Anatomy

A 10 mm port is introduced and laparoscopy performed before addressing the inguinal region. The bladder may be seen centrally with the medial umbilical folds on either side (the median umbilical fold is often not visible as it is flattened by the pneumoperitoneum). The inferior epigastric vessels lie lateral to these medial folds and are the key to laparoscopic hernia surgery. In patients with a significant layer of extraperitoneal fat they may not be immediately apparent, but must be sought carefully. The hernial defect is normally seen clearly (Figure 7.3), although small indirect sacs may not be obvious because they lie obliquely and because of the flattening effect of the pneumoperitoneum. The inguinal ligament is deep to the peritoneum and is not obvious initially. Gonadal vessels are usually visible through the peritoneum, emerging laterally to the epigastric vessels and running cranially. In men the vas may be seen at this stage; it is extraperitoneal and runs medially. The type of hernia is determined by the relationship of its neck to these structures.

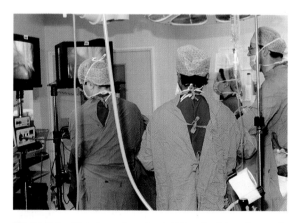

Figure 7.1 Theatre set up for left inguinal hernia repair

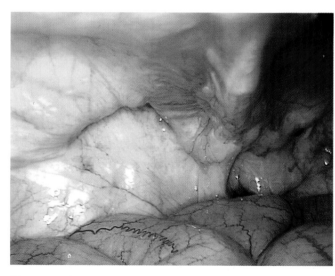

Figure 7.3 Laparoscopic view of left inguinal hernia

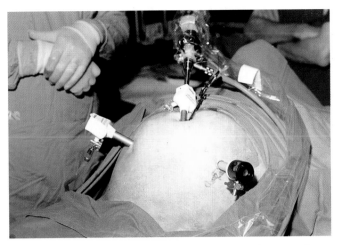

Figure 7.4 View from caudal end of patient, showing port site positions

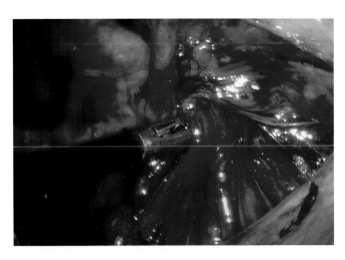

(a)

Port positions

A port is introduced in each iliac fossa at the level of, or just below, the umbilicus, taking care to avoid the epigastric vessels on the anterior abdominal wall. The size of the ports depends on the procedure: for unilateral hernia repair an ipsilateral 5 mm port and contralateral 12 mm port (for the stapling device) are required, but two 12 mm ports are optimal for bilateral hernia repair (Figure 7.4).

Hernial sac

The contents of the sac should be reduced without damaging bowel or bladder, and any adhesions should be divided. Irreducible hernias are not suitable for laparoscopic repair. On the left bowel may be stuck close to, or over, the inguinal canal and if these adhesions are congenital their division may need to be incorporated within the peritoneal dissection.

Peritoneal reflection

Scissors, preferably with diathermy, are used to incise and divide the peritoneum transversely above the inguinal ligament. Bleeding should be minimised to maximise the view and to reduce light absorption. The hernial sac may usually be reduced by grasping its apex and retracting it cranially. The peritoneal incision extends superiorly across the sac neck, from the medial umbilical fold to a point a few centimetres lateral to the inferior epigastric vessels. If the sac can not be reduced, or is large, the neck should be circumcised, preserving as much peritoneum as possible to cover the mesh. Saline may be injected into the extraperitoneal space to elevate the peritoneum by percutaneous injection from the anterior abdominal wall or under direct vision laparoscopically.[17]

Dissection

Peritoneal dissection is the same, whether the hernia is direct, indirect, or femoral and particular care should be taken with dissection across the inferior epigastric vessels. If the sac is reduced, sharp diathermy dissection and blunt pushing will aid in identifying cord structures. Inferiorly the peritoneum is elevated from the spermatic vessels and vas to prevent their inadvertent division, and peritoneal flaps are raised superiorly and inferiorly. It is possible to identify the conjoint tendon, the posterior aspect of the pubis and Cooper's ligament, the inguinal ligament (which lies more superiorly than expected),

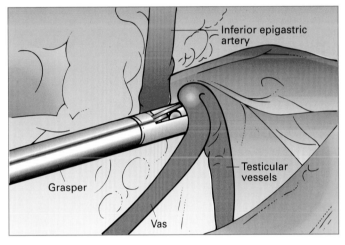

(b)

Figure 7.5 Demonstration of cord structures seen at inguinal hernia repair

cord structures, and the epigastric vessels (Figure 7.5). The danger area lies below the inguinal ligament in the angle formed between the vas and the spermatic vessels, where dissection will be over the external iliac vessels and mobilisation will take you below the inguinal ligament instead of above it. A thorough knowledge of the anatomy is essential if injury is to be avoided. Adequate dissection is important and should extend from medial to the pubic tubercle to lateral to the epigastric vessels because a good sized peritoneal flap is required (Figure 7.6). It is possible, though not necessary, to narrow the deep ring by suturing the conjoint tendon to the inguinal ligament. This may lose the benefit of a tension free repair.

Placement of the mesh

As large a mesh as possible should be used, irrespective of the size of the hernial defect. A rectangle of mesh 13 × 9 cm is usually sufficient, with the corners trimmed but not cut to shape. It is inserted through the 12 mm port and positioned in the extraperitoneal dissection. Great care should be taken to arrange the mesh to lie snugly, without rolled edges, medial to the pubic tubercle and lateral to the inferior epigastric vessels (the deep ring) with its upper margin above the conjoint tendon and its lower margin below the inguinal ligament (Figure 7.7). A combination of gentle pulling

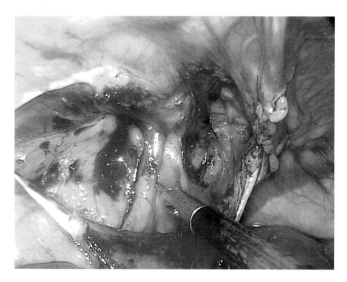

Figure 7.6 Peritoneal flaps raised over defect and cord structures

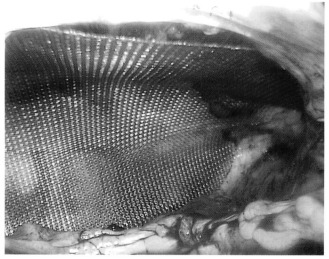

Figure 7.7 Prosthetic mesh placed over left inguinal hernia

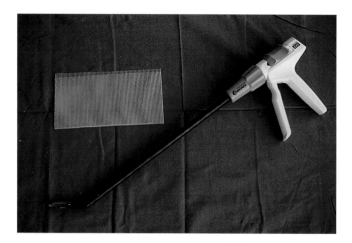

Figure 7.8 Prosthetic mesh and hernia stapling device

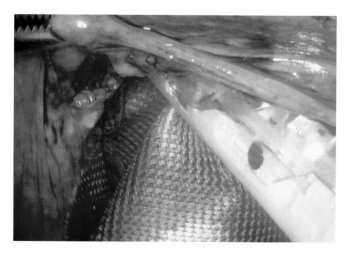

(a)

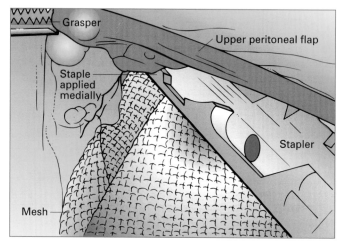

(b)

Figure 7.9 Staple being applied to mesh at medial edge of right inguinal hernia repair (near pubic tubercle)

and tapping usually achieves this. A hernia stapler (Figure 7.8) is introduced and staples inserted at the pubic tubercle/Cooper's ligament (Figure 7.9) and along the upper margin, avoiding the epigastric vessels. No attempt should be made to staple the mesh inferiorly, to avoid stapling the external iliac vessels; lateral stapling increases the risk of damaging the lateral cutaneous nerve of the thigh.

Some surgeons advocate the use of a double mesh. The first is cut laterally and placed superficial to the cord and epigastric vessels, the second is placed over the first with the vessels between the two.[18] Bilateral inguinal hernias may be repaired either using two separate meshes or by extending the medial dissection extraperitoneally across the pubis. A "bikini top" style mesh can be pulled through such that both sides are covered by the same mesh.

Peritoneal repair

The peritoneum is closed over the mesh using staples (Figure 7.10) or a running suture. At this stage the need to conserve peritoneum in the initial dissection will be appreciated. Reducing the intraperitoneal pressure to 5–6 mmHg may be helpful in reducing tension on the peritoneal flaps.

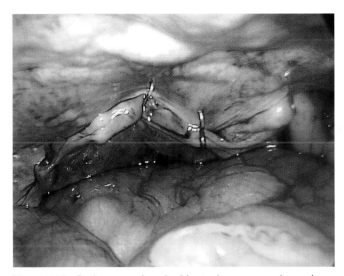

Figure 7.10 Peritoneum closed with staples over mesh repair

Intraoperative difficulties, postoperative complications

> - Pneumoperitoneum
> - Pneumoscrotum
> - Haemorrhage
> - Bladder injury
> - Neuralgia parasthetica
> - Recurrence
> - Port site herniation
> - Small bowel obstruction

Pneumoperitoneum

This may give rise to a feeling of bloatedness, which resolves in a few days. It may also produce shoulder tip pain in about 10% of patients. This will also resolve spontaneously but can be minimised by aspiration of the area above the liver at closure.[11] A pneumoscrotum may occur; this can be prevented by pressure on the scrotum at the end of the procedure or by needle venting.

Overlying bowel

Mobilisation of overlying intestine, most frequently sigmoid colon, may dictate the line of peritoneal dissection and necessitate tailoring of the relative sizes of the peritoneal flaps.

Inability to reduce the hernial sac

As in a conventional repair reduction of the sac is not an absolute necessity, and the sac may be divided. Such a manoeuvre can lead to a seroma or haematoma in the residual sac, which usually resolves spontaneously or can be aspirated 2–3 weeks later.

Haemorrhage

This is usually minor unless one of the epigastric vessels is damaged. Haemorrhage can usually be controlled using a Ligaclip or diathermy, but it may be necessary to perform a groin incision and ligate the vessels under direct vision.

Bladder injury

Several reports have documented bladder injury, which may be repaired laparoscopically,[5 18 19] although an open approach is preferred by some surgeons.[12] The repair should always be protected by the placement of a urinary catheter.

Intestinal obstruction

This has been associated with a defect in the peritoneal repair, with bowel stuck to the mesh, or with herniation through the umbilical port wound.[20]

Other complications

Postoperative urinary retention, pubic osteitis, rectus sheath haematoma or entrapment of the lateral cutaneous nerve of the thigh have all been reported.[10–12 21] Neuralgia parasthetica usually resolves within 6 weeks, but if persistent may necessitate removal of any staples from the region of the nerve.

Limitations

Laparoscopic hernia repair is not easy and involves an approach totally different from that of conventional repair, so a sound understanding of the anatomy is essential. Complications involving the bladder, bowel or mesh may turn a simple procedure into an unmitigated disaster. Such complications are rare but tend to occur early in operator experience, therefore training in the technique is essential. Landmarks may be difficult, especially in the obese. There may also be concern about the use of a synthetic material in a young patient, although this is becoming routine in the USA for conventional repair. The operating time may be reduced to 20–30 min with adequate experience.

Conclusion

Laparoscopic hernia repair embraces the anatomic and surgical principles advocated for hernia surgery by tackling the basic defect, effecting a low tension repair and avoiding disruption of the whole inguinal canal. For recurrent hernias the laparoscopic technique has much to offer and the advantages override concerns about the use of synthetic material in younger patients. The long term recurrence rate is, as yet, unknown although recurrence rates have been reported to be about 1%. Widespread uptake of this procedure should wait until the technique has been consolidated and the recurrence rates determined. Notwithstanding these constraints, the authors feel that the results will justify early enthusiasm.

1 Clinical guidelines on the management of groin hernia in adults. Report of a working party convened by the Royal College of Surgeons of England. July, 1993.
2 Serpell JW, Jarrett PEM, Johnson CD. A prospective study of bilateral hernia repair. *Ann R Coll Surg Engl* 1990;**72**:299–303.
3 Devlin HB, Gillen PHA, Waxman BP, MacNay RA. Short stay surgery for inguinal hernia: Experience of the Shouldice operation. *Br J Surg* 1986;**73**:123–4.
4 Kingsnorth AN, Nott DM, Gray MR. Prospective randomised trial comparing the Shouldice technique and plication darn for 300 inguinal hernias: a two year minimum follow-up. *Br J Surg* 1992;**79**:1068–70.
5 Capozzi JA, Berrkenfield JA, Cherry JK. Repair of inguinal hernia in the adult with prolene mesh. *Surg Gynecol Obstet* 1988;**167**:124–8.
6 Shulman AG, Amid PK, Lichtenstein IL. The safety of mesh repair for primary inguinal hernias: results of 3019 operations from five diverse surgical sources. *Am Surg* 1992;**58**:255–7.
7 Lichtenstein IL, Shulman AG, Amid PK *et al.* The pathophysiology of recurrent hernia: a new concept introducing the tension free repair. *Contemp Surg* 1989;**35**:13–18.

8 Arregui ME, Nagan RF. *Inguinal hernia: advances or controversies.* Oxford: Radcliffe Medical Press, 1994.

9 Commission on the Provision of Surgical Services. *Guidelines for day case surgery.* London: Royal College of Surgeons, 1985.

10 Newman L, Eubanks S, Mason E, Duncan TD. Is laparoscopic herniorrhaphy an effective alternative to open hernia repair. *J Laparoendosc Surg* 1993;**3**:121–8.

11 Wheeler KH. Laparoscopic inguinal herniorrhaphy with mesh: an 18 month experience. *J Laparoendosc Surg* 1993;**3**:245–50.

12 Toy FK, Snoot RT. Laparoscopic hernioplasty update. *J Laparoendosc Surg* 1992;**2**:1970–204.

13 Arregui ME, Navarrete J, Davis CJ, Nagan RF. Laparoscopic inguinal herniorrhaphy: techniques and controversies. *Surg Clin North Am* 1993;**73**:513–27.

14 Schultz L, Graber J, Pietrafitta J. Laser laparoscopic herniorrhaphy: a clinical trial, preliminary results. *J Laparoendosc Surg* 1990;**1**:41–5.

15 Filipi CJ, Fitzgibbone RJ, Salerno GM *et al.* Laparoscopic herniorrhaphy. *Surg Clin North Am* 1992;**72**:1109–24.

16 Spaw AT, Ennis BW, Spaw LP. Laparoscopic hernia repair: the anatomical basis. *J Laparoendosc Surg* 1991;**1**:269–77.

17 Dunn DC. Method of separating the peritoneal sac from the spermatic vessels during laparoscopic repair of inguinal hernia. *Br J Surg* 1993;**80**:746.

18 Felix EL, Michas C. Double-buttress laparoscopic herniorrhaphy. *J Laparoendosc Surg* 1993;**3**:1–8.

19 Font GE, Brill AI, Stuhldreher PV, Rosenzweig BA. Endoscopic management of incidental cystostomy during operative laparoscopy. *J Urol* 1993;**149**:1130–1.

20 Wegeneer ME, Chung D, Crans C, Chung D. Small bowel obstruction secondary to incarcerated Richters hernia from laparoscopic hernia repair. *J Laparoendosc Surg* 1993;**3**:173–6.

21 Eubanks S, Newman L, Goehring L *et al.* Neuralgia parasthetica: a complication of laparoscopic herniorrhaphy. *Surg Laparosc Endosc* 1993;**3**:381–5.

8 Laparoscopic appendicectomy

Timothy H Brown

Laparoscopic appendicectomy was initially described by Semm in 1983 as an incidental procedure during gynaecological laparoscopy, and he has recently outlined the technical steps involved in this operation.[1] The procedure has been performed by general surgeons since the advent and rapid implementation of laparoscopic cholecystectomy. Laparoscopic appendicectomy is now performed in the UK, Europe, Asia and the USA, though its precise role in the management of appendicitis has yet to be defined, especially as conventional appendicectomy is quick and usually straightforward, with minimal morbidity.

Indications

> • Right iliac fossa pain
> • Acute appendicitis
> • Interval appendicectomy

Perhaps the most relevant indication for laparoscopic appendicectomy is the patient who presents with right iliac fossa pain, a common surgical emergency. Some of these patients obviously have acute appendicitis but in others the diagnosis is not clear and other pathology may account for the symptoms and signs. In such patients there is an obvious advantage in being able to view the pelvis and the right iliac fossa to assess the cause of symptoms and make an accurate diagnosis. The laparoscopic approach may be employed for the therapeutic management of the presenting condition such as appendicitis, twisted or ruptured ovarian cyst, Meckel's diverticulum or salpingitis.

Advantages

> • Accurate diagnosis
> • Small wounds
> • Early mobilisation
> • Early discharge
> • Reduced wound infection

This ability to make an accurate diagnosis without recourse to a laparotomy is the biggest advantage of a laparoscopic approach to right iliac fossa pain avoiding unnecessary laparotomy or appendicectomy. There are other advantages over conventional appendicectomy. The wounds for the laparoscopic approach are three stab incisions (10 or 5 mm) rather than a longer right iliac fossa incision. The sum total length of the wounds may equal or exceed the length of the open wound, but these smaller wounds cause less discomfort and may be more acceptable cosmetically. This is certainly the case in a large patient where the right iliac fossa wound would need to be substantial (sometimes over 15 cm in length) in order to give adequate access to the peritoneal cavity. Early results would suggest that the patients have a lower requirement for postoperative analgesia, can be discharged earlier from hospital, have a lower incidence of wound infection and may return to normal activity, exercise and work significantly earlier.[2-4] However, a recent report of a randomised study of patients undergoing open or laparoscopic appendicectomy showed no significant difference as far as the postoperative course was concerned.[5]

Technical details

Operating room set up

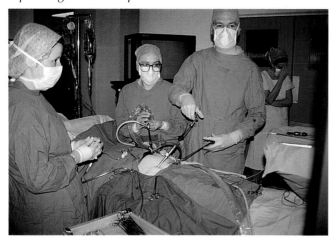

Figure 8.1 The operating room during laparoscopic appendicectomy—view from the monitor

The equipment required for laparoscopic appendicectomy is similar to that required for other laparoscopic surgery, but the placement of equipment and personnel differs. As can be seen (Figures 8.1 and 8.2), the surgeon stands on the patients left looking towards the patient's right iliac fossa. The camera operator stands on the surgeon's right and the scrub nurse on the patient's right. The video monitor is placed

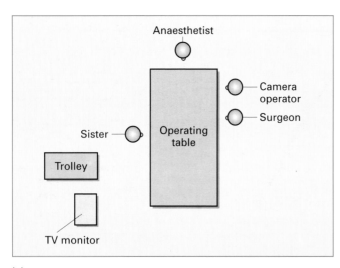

(a)

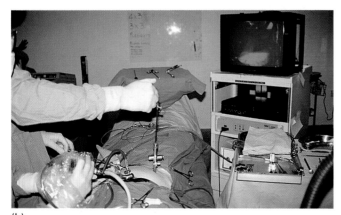

(b)

Figure 8.2 (a) Plan of operating room set up; (b) set up, shown from the head of the patient

slightly to the right of the patient's feet with the instrument trolley also on the right side of the patient. Positioning of the diathermy and suction and irrigation apparatus should be at the convenience of the operating staff.

Placement of ports

Three ports are required for a laparoscopic appendicectomy; reusable or disposable ports may be used. The Veress needle is inserted just below the umbilicus and inflation commenced after testing for correct placement. A 10 mm port is inserted below the umbilicus and two further 10 mm ports are placed under vision, one in the right and one in the left iliac fossa (Figure 8.3). Some surgeons also place a port in the suprapubic area or the right upper quadrant in order to manipulate the appendix, but this is not routinely required.

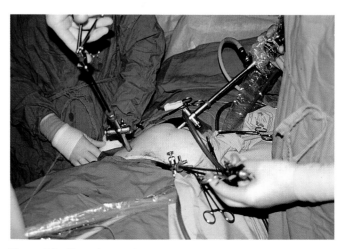

Figure 8.3 Port sites at the umbilicus, right iliac fossa and left iliac fossa for laparoscopic appendicectomy

Operative procedure

After inflation of the peritoneal cavity the laparoscope is introduced and the peritoneum surveyed. The operating table may be adjusted to achieve better visualisation of the appendix, usually by performing head down and right side up tilt. The right iliac fossa and pelvis are inspected to confirm the diagnosis and if an appendicectomy is to be performed the position of the two operating ports are determined by the position of the appendix. At this stage a small amount of saline with heparin may be introduced to prevent clotting of any haemorrhage, thus enabling blood to be aspirated more easily. The appendix is identified and retracted away from the caecum and terminal ileum (Figure 8.4). The more inflamed the appendix the more difficult this procedure can be, and the technique may need to vary if the appendix lies retrocaecally. The appendix and its mesentery are held by a pair of forceps introduced via the right iliac fossa port, and an incision is made across the mesentery towards the appendix using diathermy or sharp dissection. Before the incision is made clips can be placed across the mesenteric vessels, or across the mesentery itself if the vessels are not visible (Figure 8.5), the mesoappendix is fat or there is inflammation present. Any obvious windows of mesentery between the branches of the appendicular artery can be opened and the vessel clipped between them using endoscopically placed clips or a preformed

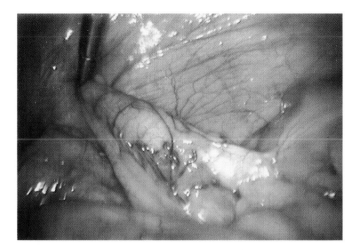

Figure 8.4 The appendix is grasped and retracted away from the caecum

slip knot. The mesoappendix and the appendix are separated by diathermy and dissection to leave a skeletalised appendix down to its base at the caecum. At this stage the mesoappendix may be further secured using a preformed slip knot.

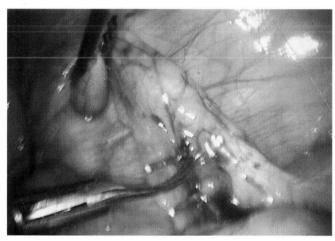

(a)

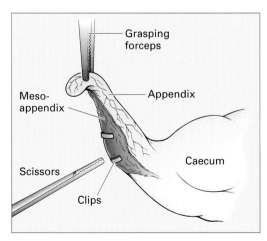

(b)

Figure 8.5 The mesoappendix can be clipped and divided

Appendix division and removal

Division and removal of the appendix may be achieved by one of three approaches.

Laparoscopically assisted appendicectomy

This technique[6] is rarely used. It involves manipulation of the appendix into the right iliac fossa 10 mm port with subsequent traction of the caecum to the anterior abdominal wall. The port is removed leaving the appendix outside the abdominal cavity with the caecum visible through the wound. An appendicectomy may now be performed with ligation of the base, amputation of the appendix and burial of the stump using a pursestring suture. The caecum is returned to the peritoneal cavity and the port reinserted for inspection, to irrigate the peritoneal cavity and to aspirate any collected fluid. The disadvantages of this technique are bringing the appendix up to the abdominal wall, and the risk of wound infection with direct contact between the appendix and the skin.

Endoloop ligation of the appendix

This is the most commonly employed technique.[27] Once the appendix is separated from its mesentery down to the caecum, an Endoloop (Ethicon Endosurgery, Edinburgh, UK) is introduced via the left iliac fossa port. This loop is backloaded into a reducing port (with the loop distally) and the reducing port is placed into the 10 mm port, allowing the loop to be advanced into the peritoneal cavity. The forceps holding the appendix are opened to release the appendix and are directed through the loop to grasp the appendix again. The loop is manipulated to the base of the appendix, the external portion of the Endoloop is snapped, and the knot pusher advanced to tighten the Roeder knot around the base of the appendix (Figure 8.6). The outer end of the ligature is then divided, the pusher extracted, a pair of scissors introduced and the Endoloop divided just above the knot. This procedure is repeated with a second loop, which is placed just distal to the first knot. A third Endoloop is introduced via the right iliac fossa port with the forceps exchanged to the left iliac fossa port. The loop is placed about 5 mm distal to the second loop along the appendix, and the appendix is divided between the second and third loops (Figure 8.7). The pusher is withdrawn and the appendix may then be removed by pulling on the third Endoloop. The appendix is retracted into the reducing port (Figure 8.8) and the port and appendix removed together, thus avoiding contamination of the skin. A clip can be placed across the appendix instead of the third Endoloop. The stump of the

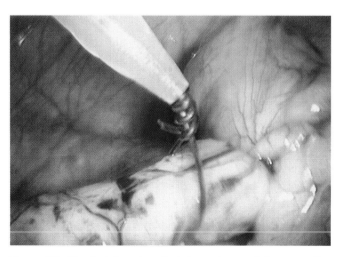

Figure 8.6 The Endoloop knot is tightened around the appendix base

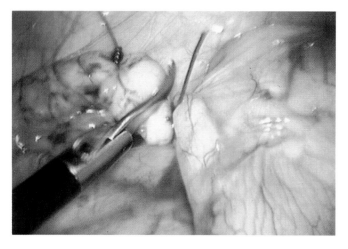

Figure 8.7 The appendix is divided between the second and third Endoloops

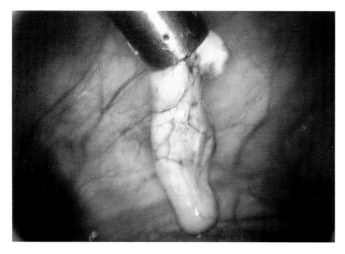

Figure 8.8 The appendix is extracted through the port

appendix (Figure 8.9) is irrigated and diathermied and the right iliac fossa is irrigated with antibiotic solution, which is then aspirated. After checking for adequate haemostasis the CO_2 and ports are removed and the wounds closed.

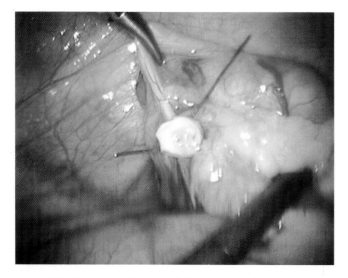

Figure 8.9 The appendix stump is inspected and may be irrigated with saline

Appendicectomy using an endoscopic stapler
Using this technique the base of the appendix, with or without its adjoining mesoappendix, can be clipped and divided using a stapler (for example, Endo-GIA, Autosuture) introduced via a 12 mm port in the left iliac fossa to divide and staple each side of the appendix, thus preventing spillage. It is a more expensive technique than Endoloop ligation but may be especially useful in a patient with retrocaecal appendicitis, in whom the appendix can be resected in a retrograde fashion after the appendix base has been divided.

With either of the second two techniques the stump of the appendix is not buried although the tip can be diathermied. It is possible to bury the stump using intracorporeal suturing but this is technically difficult, prolongs the operative time and has been shown not to add any benefit when performed in conventional appendicectomy.[8]

Difficulties and complications

- Perforation of the appendix base
- Haemorrhage
- Spillage of pus/appendicular contents
- Extracting the appendix

Perforation of the appendix base
In the second two techniques described above perforation of the appendix makes the application of an Endoloop or Endo-GIA stapler difficult or impossible. In such a situation it may be better to suture the base of the appendix rather than ligate it, elevate the caecum to the right iliac fossa port and close the appendix base through the skin incision, or convert to an open procedure.

Haemorrhage
This may occur from the mesoappendix, from inflammatory tissue, or from an abscess cavity around an acutely inflamed appendix. As in all laparoscopic surgery it is vital to identify the source of the bleeding and, because of the magnification obtained using the video systems, it is usually possible to identify a vessel or an area of blood loss. Haemostasis can be achieved by grasping the bleeding point with a pair of forceps and applying diathermy, ligating with an Endoloop or applying a clip. Hook or ball diathermy may be used in an area of oozing, but care must be taken not to damage the bowel wall. Tamponade of the bleeding area can be achieved using a pledget held in a pair of grasping forceps. If the haemorrhage is uncontrollable, conversion to open appendicectomy is the only option.

Spillage of pus or appendicular contents
Although spillage introduces infected material into the peritoneal cavity this can be irrigated with saline (with an antibiotic if required) and aspirated. The patient should be treated with an antibiotic regimen similar to that used for open appendicectomy. The risk of intra-abdominal abscess formation does not seem to be increased, and the wound infection rate is probably reduced with a laparoscopic procedure.[3]

Extracting the appendix

Occasionally the appendix is too bulky to remove safely through a 10 mm port, especially if some of the mesoappendix is attached. The first approach in such a case would be to place the appendix in a "Bert" bag (Vernon Carus, Preston, UK) before extraction, as this will enable more traction to be applied than pulling on the appendix itself. If the appendix can not be removed this way it may be extracted along with the port, or the port dilated to a size through which the appendix can be removed. Ideally, the appendix should be removed without contact with the skin edge, but if contamination does occur thorough irrigation of the wound should reduce the risk of postoperative wound infection.

Applicability

The cosmetic appearance following laparoscopic appendicectomy is excellent, with a smaller scar than

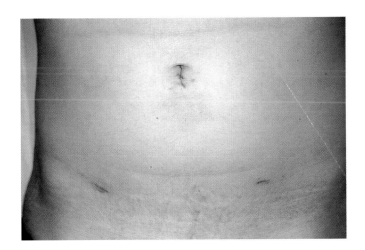

Figure 8.10 Postoperative scars of laparoscopic appendicectomy are much less significant than those achieved using conventional techniques

that achieved by most conventional appendicectomies (Figure 8.10). The main advantages with the laparoscopic approach are smaller wounds, earlier mobilisation, earlier discharge, and a reduction in wound infection.[3] These should be especially beneficial to the older patient and to the patient who is overweight, in whom a conventional wound may need to be substantial. For the child or the young thin adult the advantages may not be as obvious because the cumulative wound size, time to mobilisation, time to discharge and the time to return to normal life may be similar to that of the open approach. The main benefit in such patients is the accurate diagnosis possible with the laparoscopic approach, which should avoid unnecessary laparotomy or appendicectomy. I believe that the role of laparoscopic appendicectomy in the management of patients with right iliac fossa pain or appendicitis has still to be clearly defined, but would recommend this approach where the diagnosis is in doubt, or where the scar from an open approach would be large.

Acknowledgements

The author is grateful to Stryker UK, and particularly to Mr B D Cleaver for the intraoperative illustrations in Figures 4, 5, 6, 7, 8 and 9.

1 Semm K, Freys I. Endoscopic appendectomy: technical operative steps. *Min Invasive Ther* 1991;1:41–50.
2 Pier A, Gotz F, Bacher C, Ibald R. Laparoscopic Appendectomy. *World J Surg* 1993;17:29–33.
3 Lujan-Mompean JA, Robles-Campos R, Parrilla-Paricio P, Soria-Aledo V, Garcia-Ayllon J. Laparoscopic versus open appendicectomy: a prospective assessment. *Br J Surg* 1994;81:133–5.
4 Schroder DM, Lathrop JC, Lloyd CR, Boccaccio JE, Hawasli A. Laparoscopic appendectomy for acute appendicitis. *Am Surg* 1993;59:541–8.
5 Tate JJ, Dawson JW, Chung SC, Lau WY, Li AK. Laparoscopic versus open appendicectomy: prospective randomised trial. *Lancet* 1993;342:633–7.
6 Byrne DS, Bell G, Morrice JJ, Orr G. Technique for laparoscopic appendicectomy. *Br J Surg* 1992;79:574–5.
7 Saye WB, Rives DA, Cochran EB. Laparoscopic Appendectomy: 3 years' experience. *Surg Laparosc Endosc* 1991;1:109–15.
8 Engstrom L, Fenyo G. Appendicectomy: assessment of stump invagination versus simple ligation. a prospective randomised trial. *Br J Surg* 1985;72:971–2.

9 Laparoscopy for upper gastrointestinal disorders

Timothy H Brown, John Bancewicz

The techniques employed in minimal access surgery for biliary disease have been applied in other areas of surgery, especially hernia repair, appendicectomy, and the treatment of benign gastro-oesophageal disease. Patients with benign gastro-oesophageal disease are usually of an age where the advantages of reduced postoperative pain, early discharge and early return to work outweigh the increased time required to perform laparoscopic surgery. As the procedures used to treat benign gastro-oesophageal disease (see below) are more difficult to perform laparoscopically and because they are used in treating non-malignant disease it is essential that the appropriate procedure is selected and that the surgeon is adequately trained in the wider aspects of oesophagogastric surgery. There is a danger that an inappropriate procedure may be undertaken because the patient has been inadequately assessed, or that an appropriate procedure may be performed by a poorly trained surgeon.

A number of conditions classified under benign gastro-oesophageal disease can be treated using laparoscopic techniques. These fall into three groups: gastro-oesophageal reflux disease, achalasia and oesophageal motility problems, and complicated peptic ulcer disease.

- Nissen fundoplication
- Heller's myotomy
- Highly selective vagotomy
- Posterior vagotomy and anterior seromyotomy
- Perforated duodenal ulcer repair

Gastro-oesophageal reflux disease

This is a common complaint, as many patients suffer from acid reflux, regurgitation, or heartburn. Most can be managed conservatively by altering their lifestyle (weight loss, raising the head end of bed, etc) or with medication (such as antacids, H_2 receptor blockers, proton pump inhibitors). Surgery should be considered only in patients who continue to be symptomatic despite treatment, or who do not wish to take medication for an extended period of time. In such patients thorough preoperative assessment is essential.

Preoperative assessment

In patients with a history suggesting gastro-oesophageal reflux disease the diagnosis is made using the following techniques.

- Oesophagogastroduodenoscopy
- 24 hour pH monitoring
- Oesophageal manometry
- Contrast radiology

Endoscopy is essential to assess oesophagitis, hiatal hernia, and Barrett's oesophagus. Oesophageal manometry and 24 hour pH monitoring confirm the diagnosis in a measurable way and exclude other conditions with similar symptomatology. Contrast studies may be needed to produce good anatomical information. Once the diagnosis is confirmed and the decision made that surgical intervention is appropriate, the patient is submitted for surgery. The surgical procedure of choice is a Nissen fundoplication,[1] or a modification of this technique. The aim of this procedure is to increase the length of intra-abdominal oesophagus and to increase the effectiveness of the lower oesophageal sphincter. The procedure involves wrapping the fundus of the stomach around the distal oesophagus to prevent the reflux of acid fluid from the stomach into the distal oesophagus.

Nissen fundoplication

Positioning

The patient is placed supine on the operating table with the legs in Lloyd Davies stirrups. This enables the table to be rotated until the patient is tilted at an angle of 30°, facing the surgeon. The first assistant stands on the patient's left and the second assistant (camera holder) stands on the patient's right (Figure 9.1). The surgeon stands in the space between the patient's legs.[2] The nurse and instrument trolley are placed behind and to the surgeon's right.

The Veress needle is introduced just below the umbilicus and the peritoneal cavity inflated. A 10 mm port is positioned between the umbilicus and the xiphisternum, the laparoscope is introduced via this port and four other ports placed under direct vision in the positions shown in Figure 9.2. The port under the right costal margin is for the liver retractor and for the

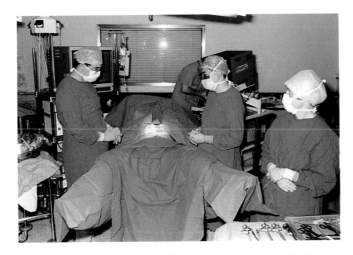

Figure 9.1 Position of patient for laparoscopic fundoplication

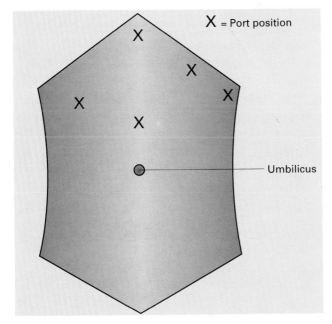

Figure 9.2 Position of ports for laparoscopic fundoplication

forceps, which pass behind the oesophagus. The epigastric port, close to the xiphisternum, is used for forceps for manipulation, or a liver retractor when required. The more cephalad of the left costal ports is used for forceps, scissors and needle holder, and the more caudal for Babcock's forceps for gastric retraction. Suction and irrigation may be introduced via any of the ports as required. All five ports need to be 10 mm in diameter, and fixing devices make their use easier.

Fundal mobilisation

The left hepatic lobe is elevated, the fundus identified and gently retracted using non-crushing clamps or forceps. The stomach may then be manipulated to stretch the short gastric vessels, which are freed from connective tissue, clipped and divided. Two clips are placed on the splenic side of the vessels to reduce the risk of the clip slipping and haemorrhage. Once the epigastric vessels have been divided up to the gastro-oesophageal junction the fundus is mobilised to enable a posterior wrap around the oesophagus. In patients who have recently lost weight the fundus may be adequately mobile for a wrap without dividing the short gastric vessels, and some surgeons advocate a fundus wrap

without dividing the short gastric vessels as a routine. Whichever technique is used, the wrap must be free of tension or the fundoplication will tend to unwrap.

Oesophageal mobilisation

The hiatus and distal oesophagus is now cleared. The right and left margins of the hiatus are identified and freed from surrounding tissue to expose the right and

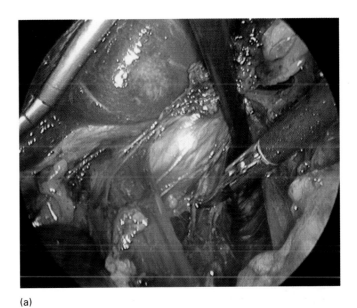

(a)

(b)

Figure 9.3 Laparoscopic view of crura and oesophagus

left crural muscles (Figure 9.3). The oesophagus is cleared until it can be gently elevated and moved laterally. Great care must be taken when handling the oesophagus as it may be friable, particularly in a patient with oesophagitis. Clearing some of the lesser curve of the stomach at this stage helps to identify the crura and the oesophagus. After the oesophagus has been freed forceps are passed from the patient's right between the oesophagus and the crura to pull the fundus behind the oesophagus. Care must be taken not to pass the forceps blindly behind the oesophagus to avoid oesophageal damage.

Hiatus closure

The size of the hiatus should be assessed and the crura sutured together if necessary. However, the hiatus must allow the oesophagus containing a 50 Fr mercury bougie to pass through the crura and still have space for a 10 mm rod. The needle is introduced through the left crus (Figure 9.4) and then passed through the right crus before ligation. The hiatus is closed using non-absorbable sutures (such as Gore-tex), which are tied externally. The knot is directed down using a knot pusher after each throw. Gore-tex allows easy extracorporeal ligation and causes a suitable tissue reaction. A small patch of Teflon placed on each side of the tissue before ligation of the suture will prevent the Gore-tex cutting through the tissue (Figure 9.5). It is easier to assess the tension on a knot tied like this than one tied internally.

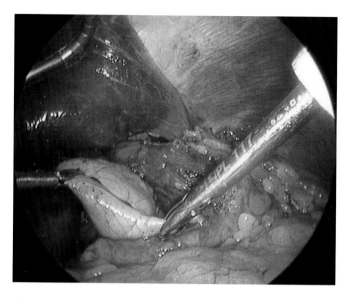

Figure 9.6 Fundus wrap pulled posterior to the oesophagus

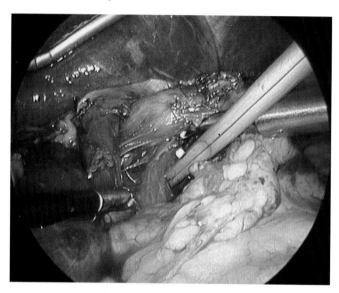

Figure 9.4 Placement of needle through left crus

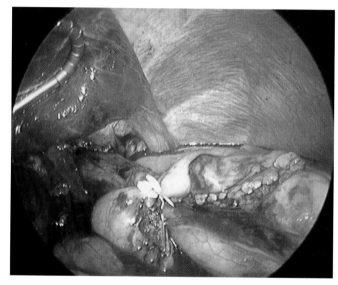

(a)

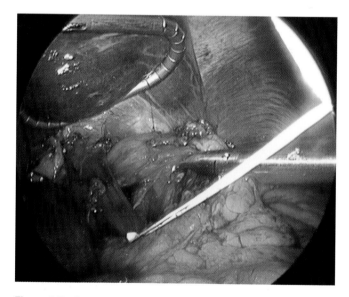

Figure 9.5 Gore-tex knot tightened to close hiatus. Note the Teflon patch, to prevent the Gore-tex cutting through tissue

Forming the wrap

The freed fundus is then grasped and gently pulled behind the oesophagus (Figure 9.6) using Babcock's forceps or bowel grasping forceps. Care must be taken to avoid avulsing clips as the fundus is retracted. The

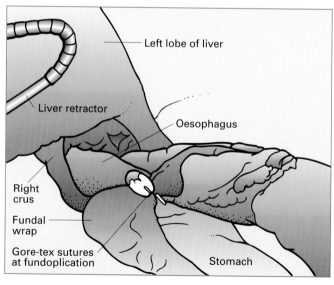

(b)

Figure 9.7 Nissen fundoplication, wrap in place

fundus is pulled through without tension and should remain in place when released from the forceps. The wrap is made around a 50 mm mercury bougie, with enough space to pass a 10 mm rod between the wrap and the gastric wall. The length of the suture line will be 1–1·5 cm. This "floppy" Nissen will give the best combination of a low "unwrap rate", a low incidence of postoperative complications (dysphagia, gas bloat), and a low recurrence of reflux symptoms. The first suture is passed through the fundus on the left, through the muscle at the cardia and though the wrap on the right. This will help to maintain the position of the wrap and prevent it from slipping into the chest, or onto the body of the stomach. A further 2–3 sutures are placed along the wrap, approximating the two edges of the wrap without excessive tension. A second row of sutures is placed superficial to the initial row to reinforce the wrap (Figure 9.7).

The combination of use of a non-absorbable suture material, two layers of sutures, wrap of 1–1·5 cm, and a "floppy" Nissen reduces the unwrap rate.

Closure

The peritoneal cavity is irrigated, the fluid aspirated and a further assessment of the fundoplication made. The CO_2 is released, the ports removed and the abdominal wall defects closed.

Complications

Postoperative pain is reduced, which allows early mobilisation, discharge and return to normal activities. There may be a slight increase in initial dysphagia. Long term effectiveness of this procedure must be assessed after at least 6 months.

The major risk of this procedure is perforation of the oesophagus, as finger assessment of its friability and position is not possible. Great care must be taken in handling the oesophagus, and mobilisation must not be undertaken blindly. A suspicion of perforation should be checked with gastroscopy and immediately repaired. Death can occur from oesophageal perforation.

Achalasia

Achalasia consists of an aperistaltic oesophagus coupled to a high pressure lower oesophageal sphincter. The combined effects of this condition are a tight lower oesophageal sphincter and a grossly dilated proximal oesophagus. The management of achalasia involves careful assessment, to confirm the diagnosis and exclude less common conditions with similar symptoms. Endoscopy and manometry will exclude other conditions and confirm the diagnosis of achalasia; and 24 h pH monitoring may be used to exclude reflux disease.

Achalasia is treated by transoesophageal balloon dilatation. A balloon is passed down the oesophagus to the lower oesophageal sphincter under radiological screening and is inflated with fluid containing dye. A high pressure is maintained for 1 minute, to disrupt the lower oesophageal sphincter. This procedure may be repeated if the first attempt is unsuccessful, but if two attempts fail then surgery is required. This surgery consists of a myotomy of the distal oesophagus (Heller's procedure) which may be performed laparoscopically[3] or thoracoscopically.[4]

Laparoscopic Heller's myotomy

The patient's position and the port placements are the same as for Nissen fundoplication. The stomach is grasped by Babcock's forceps and distracted from the hiatus. The tissue anterior to the oesophagus is divided with a combination of sharp, blunt and diathermy dissection until the oesophagus is seen clearly in the peritoneal cavity and into the posterior mediastinum. The posterior attachments of the oesophagus and cardia are left intact to prevent postoperative reflux. The cardia is displayed and its fat pad identified and removed. The seromuscular surface of the distal oesophagus and cardia may then be identified and the oesophageal muscle is divided longitudinally for 5 cm, and for 1 cm onto the stomach. The muscle is separated using forceps and pledget dissection until the oesophageal mucosa bulges between the fibres. A gastroscope is passed to ensure that these fibres are adequately divided to allow easy passage across the cardia, and that the mucosa has not been breached. Haemostasis is checked, the peritoneal cavity irrigated and fluid aspirated, and the CO_2 and ports are removed.

This procedure may be performed without a covering fundoplication (often required with an open Heller's myotomy).

Peptic ulcer disease

Peptic ulcer disease is common, but it is rare for a patient to require surgery unless complications arise. A few patients do not respond to medical treatment, are unable to continue with medical treatment, are non-compliant, or develop a complication of the disease. In these patients antiulcer surgery is justifiable. Surgery may be an acceptable alternative to continued conservative treatment, long term antiulcer therapy, or recurrent attacks of disease.

There are two main approaches to laparoscopic antiulcer surgery: highly selective vagotomy or posterior vagotomy and seromyotomy. Some surgeons continue to advocate a truncal vagotomy and pyloroplasty, but this procedure is no longer used by many gastric surgeons because of its long term morbidity.

Highly selective vagotomy

Laparoscopic highly selective vagotomy[5] is performed as in open surgery, with the patient's position and the placement of the ports similar to that used for laparoscopic fundoplication. Babcock's forceps are placed via a left sided port to grasp the greater curve of the stomach and to retract it laterally and caudally. The lesser curve of the stomach is put on stretch to show the anterior nerve of Laterjet. The oesophagus is identified and cleared and slung with nylon tape, which allows the surgeon to swing the oesophagus to the right, the left, or to elevate it as required to clear the posterior surface of the oesophagus of vagal fibres. The anterior nerve of Laterjet is also slung with a nylon tape and retracted towards the liver to protect it from inadvertent damage. The nerves and vessels between the nerve of Laterjet and the lesser curve of the stomach are divided with scissors, diathermy or clips—this requires care and must not be rushed. Dissection proceeds in both longitudinal and posterior directions along the lesser curve to the "crow's foot" of nerve branches just beyond the incisura, and posteriorly into the lesser sac. These nerves are divided carefully and haemostasis secured. The distal 6–8 cm of the oesophagus is cleared of vagal fibres; this is assisted by retracting the angle of His using Babcock's forceps or a nylon sling. It is particularly important that the nerve of Grassi, in the left lateral peritoneal reflection of the angle of His, is divided. This procedure may be slow and tedious, but care at this stage will result in a good outcome as far as decreased acid output is concerned.

The procedure is finished once the anterior and posterior nerves of Laterjet have been separated from the lesser sac of the stomach. The completeness of vagotomy may be tested during the operation. The peritoneal cavity is irrigated and aspirated, the CO_2 released, and ports withdrawn. The effectiveness of the procedure may be assessed with formal testing or by long term follow up studies.

Posterior vagotomy and seromyotomy

Many surgeons find highly selective vagotomy time consuming and difficult, and its efficacy is very operator-dependent. The Taylor procedure[6] consists of posterior truncal vagotomy coupled with selective vagotomy, achieved by dividing the nerves of the seromuscular layer of the anterior gastric wall (Figure 9.8). This appeals to

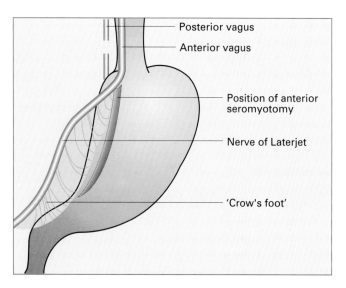

Figure 9.8 Taylor's procedure—posterior vagotomy and anterior seromyotomy

Labels in figure: Posterior vagus; Anterior vagus; Position of anterior seromyotomy; Nerve of Laterjet; 'Crow's foot'

a wider group of surgeons as it achieves an outcome similar to that of highly selective vagotomy, without requiring the length of time or difficult dissection. This procedure has been used laparoscopically with good early results.[7]

The patient is positioned and the ports placed as for the Nissen fundoplication. The posterior vagus is approached adjacent to the lesser curve of the stomach near the cardia, where the tissue is incised and the posterior vagus identified posterior to the oesophagus and medial to the right crus. It is cleared and divided between clips or diathermied, and a section removed. The anterior aspect of the stomach is put on stretch and an incision made from the oesophagus to the incisura parallel to and 1·5 cm from the lesser curve.[7] Diathermy is used to mark this line and to cut through the serosa, and the muscular layers are separated by forceps or pledget dissection until the mucosa bulges between the muscle layers: this is similar to the technique of Heller's myotomy. Diathermy is used for more major bundles of

muscle fibres and for controlling haemorrhage. It is important that the mucosa remains intact; this can be tested by inflating the stomach via a nasogastric tube. After completing the seromyotomy the incision is closed by a running suture along its length to overlap its two borders and prevent the nerve fibres regrowing. Haemostasis is secured, the area is irrigated and aspirated, the CO_2 released, and ports are removed.

Emergency treatment of perforated duodenal ulcer

Complications of peptic ulceration continue to occur, and some (such as perforated duodenal ulcer) may be managed using a laparoscopic approach.

- Omental patch
- Gelatine sponge and fibrin sealant with or without omental patch
- Omental plug with or without fibrin sealant

One technique involves the initial port being placed under the umbilicus and the diagnosis confirmed. Peritoneal lavage is necessary to help to clear intraperitoneal soiling. The perforation is almost always on the anterior surface of the first part of the duodenum and is easily seen. Two further ports are placed under direct vision to the right and left of the midline, their exact location depending on the position of the perforation.

The next step is to grasp a piece of omentum and move it to the perforation. A suture is placed through healthy duodenum and passed out through the perforation, then back through the perforation and out through healthy antrum. This suture is ligated around the omental patch placed over the perforation.[8] More than one suture may be required. A stapling device has been used to tack the omental patch down onto the healthy duodenum, antrum and falciform ligament.[9]

A second technique includes the use of a gelatine sponge plug placed into the perforation and sealed with fibrin sealant,[10] used with, or without, an omental patch.[11] It is possible to suture an omental patch over the perforation[12] but this can be technically difficult because it requires intracorporeal suturing and knot tying.

A third approach[13] involves identifying the perforation. A nasogastric tube is then passed into the stomach and directed out through the perforation into the peritoneal cavity, with the assistance of the operating surgeon. A piece of omentum is attached to the end of the nasogastric tube with chromic catgut and the nasogastric tube withdrawn into the stomach, plugging the perforation with omentum. The seal can be reinforced by serosal sutures, or by dripping fibrin glue onto the omental plug and observing until it is sealed. The catgut suture will dissolve within a few days and allow the nasogastric tube to be removed.

Acknowledgements

The authors are grateful to the Medical Illustration Department of Hope Hospital, Salford, for Figure 1 and for the use of Stryker equipment for the intraoperative views in Figures 3–7.

1 Dallemagne B, Weerts JM, Jehaes C, Markiewicz S, Lombard R. Laparoscopic Nissen fundoplication: preliminary report. *Surg Laparosc Endosc* 1991;**1**:138–43.

2 Cadiere GB, Houben JJ, Bruyns J, Himpens J, Panzer JM, Gelin M. Laparoscopic Nissen fundoplication: technique and preliminary results. *Br J Surg* 1994;**81**:400–3.

3 Shimi S, Nathanson L, Cuschieri A. Laparoscopic cardiomyotomy for achalasia. *J R Coll Surg Edinb* 1991;**36**:152–4.

4 Manson JRT, Darzi A, Carey PD, Guillou PJ. Thorascopic Heller's cardiomyotomy: a new approach for achalasia. *Surg Laparosc Endosc* 1994; **4**:6–8.

5 Dallemagne B, Weerts JM, Jehaes C, Markiewicz S, Lombard R. Laparoscopic highly selective vagotomy. *Br J Surg* 1994;**81**:554–6.

6 Taylor TV, Gunn AA, Macleod DAD, MacLellan I. Anterior lesser curve seromyotomy and posterior truncal vagotomy in the treatment of chronic duodenal ulcer. *Lancet* 1982;**ii**:846–8.

7 Mouiel J, Katkhouda N. Laparoscopic vagotomy for chronic duodenal ulcer disease. *World J Surg* 1993;**17**:34–9.

8 Sunderland GT, Chisholm EM, Lau WY, Chung SCS, Li AKC. Laparoscopic repair of perforated peptic ulcer. *Br J Surg* 1992;**79**:785.

9 Darzi A, Cheshire NJ, Somers SS, Super PA, Guillou PJ, Monson JRT. Laparoscopic omental patch repair of perforated duodenal ulcer with an automated stapler. *Br J Surg* 1993;**80**:1552.

10 Tate JJT, Dawson JW, Lau WY, Li AKC. Sutureless laparoscopic treatment of perforated duodenal ulcer. *Br J Surg* 1993;**80**:235.

11 Mouret P, Francois Y, Vignal J, Barth X, Lombard-Plaket R. Laparoscopic treatment of perforated peptic ulcer. *Br J Surg* 1990;**77**:1006.

12 Isaac J, Tekant Y, Kiong KC, Ngoi SS, Goh P. Laparoscopic repair of perforated duodenal ulcer. *Gastrointest Endosc* 1994;**40**:68–9.

13 Karanjia ND, Shanahan DJ, Knight MJ. Omental patching of a large perforated duodenal ulcer: a new method. *Br J Surg* 1993;**80**:65.

10 Laparoscopic colorectal surgery

D D Kerrigan, N R Hulton

Laparoscopic cholecystectomy, herniorrhaphy and appendicectomy have allowed many surgeons to consolidate their laparoscopic skills to a point where attention has now focused on developing these techniques to allow more complex, major surgery. Unfortunately the rush to implement laparoscopic colorectal surgery without careful critical appraisal has once again obscured the key issues. The question is not whether these procedures are technically possible (they undoubtedly are) but whether they confer any advantage over conventional surgery. If they do, which patients are most likely to benefit, and are there any individuals in whom a minimal access approach would be detrimental?

Potential advantages

- Less ileus
- Shorter hospital stay
- Better cosmesis
- Reduced risk of incisional hernia
- Patient acceptability
- Reduced postoperative pain
- Earlier mobilisation
- Reduced risk of venous thrombosis, or pulmonary embolism
- Reduced incidence of chest infection, or septic complications

Potential disadvantages

- Abdominal wall seeding of cancer cells
- Prolonged operating time
- Expensive equipment, lagging behind technical requirements
- Incision may be needed for specimen retrieval and anastomosis
- Difficulty in localising tumours
- ? Less radical cancer resections
- ? Not suitable for emergency resections

Basic principles

Basic surgical principles must be adhered to. Excellent exposure of the operative field with adequate visualisation of vital structures, careful near bloodless dissection, and avoidance of peritoneal contamination with tumour or enteric contents are essential. Similarly the extent of bowel mobilisation, the level at which the vascular pedicles are ligated, and the levels of resection should reflect those of the traditional operation as closely as possible. Anastomoses must be tension free and well vascularised. Any compromise of these basic principles is unacceptable and if doubt exists conversion to an open operation is mandatory.

Indications

Colectomy for benign disease:
- Inflammatory bowel disease
- Benign polyps
- Polyposis coli
- Diverticulosis
- Slow transit constipation

Colectomy for malignant disease:
- Abdominoperineal resection
- Palliative resection

Other indications:
- Rectopexy
- Ileostomy/colostomy
- Reversal of Hartmann's procedure
- Sigmoid myotomy
- Preoperative staging

Minimal access segmental or total colectomy is possible and has been applied in patients with inflammatory bowel disease, colonic adenomas unsuitable for endoscopic snaring, polyposis coli, diverticular disease, slow transit constipation and other benign conditions.[1]

There is no reason why a minimal access approach could not be used in the formation of a trephine colostomy, an ileostomy or even to assist in reversal of Hartmann's procedure. Techniques for carrying out laparoscopic rectopexy have also been described; this could be a useful option in elderly patients if prolapse is not associated with constipation.

Relative contraindications

> - Emergency surgery
> - Most colorectal cancers unless part of trial
> - Obesity
> - Suboptimal equipment and assistance
> - Chronic obstructive airways disease (pneumoperitoneum, CO_2 retention)
> - Coagulopathy

It would seem unwise to carry out major bowel resections in emergency cases such as perforated diverticulum, toxic megacolon or large bowel obstruction. Patients who are obese can also be problematic, particularly when it comes to identifying major vessels during division of the mesocolon. Surprisingly, a history of previous abdominal surgery does not appear to increase the rate of conversion to open surgery.[2] Because a large incision is required to retrieve bulky specimens, patients with such tumours are probably best treated conventionally.

Malignant disease

Resections performed for malignant disease are controversial.[3] A recent publication[4] has highlighted an increasing number of port site metastatic deposits (sometimes away from the site of tumour removal), which gives great cause for concern regarding laparoscopic surgery for malignant disease. In view of this, with the exception of palliative resections, minimal access colorectal cancer surgery should be carried out only as part of randomised trials comparing laparoscopic and conventional surgery.

Although mesenteric lymph node counts are reportedly similar in open and laparoscopic resections,[2] this is a notoriously unreliable guide to the adequacy of surgery. We do not yet know whether cancer patients treated laparoscopically have received adequate treatment. In the USA the American Association of Colorectal Surgeons has introduced a register containing details of all those who have undergone minimal access colorectal surgery. A similar prospective audit of British surgeons and their patients is urgently required.

However, one radical cancer operation is eminently suitable to the laparoscopic approach: abdominoperineal resection (APR). Laparoscopic mobilisation of the healthy left colon and rectum down to the levators, with intracorporeal division of the vascular pedicles and bowel, avoids the requirement for an abdominal incision. The operation is usually completed within 3 h by removing the specimen through a standard perineal incision, which does not compromise local cancer clearance. The stoma can be brought out through an enlarged left iliac fossa port site. To date there is only one reported case of recurrence at the port site after laparoscopically assisted APR. This occurred at the sites of a surgical drain. It has been suggested that the use of pelvic and wound lavage with cancericidal agents may ameliorate this rare complication.[4]

Technical details

Preparation

Preoperative preparation is identical to that for the open procedure. Following induction of general anaesthesia a urinary catheter is passed, and the patient placed in the Lloyd Davies position (a nasogastric tube may be in place). Access to the anus is important as tactile sensation within the peritoneal cavity is lost, and it may be necessary to introduce an endoscope to identify the site of the lesion (Figure 10.1). Endoscopic injection of India ink or methylene blue into the bowel wall at the site of the disease may be helpful (Figure 10.2). Some surgeons insist on performing a preoperative barium enema to aid accurate localisation of the tumour. Others have performed preoperative colonoscopy and marked the lesion by injection of charcoal into the bowel wall.

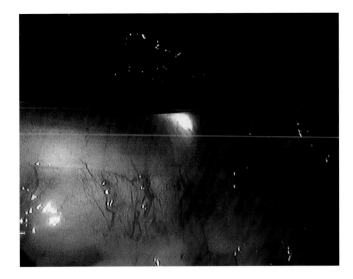

Figure 10.1 Colonoscope transilluminating bowel at site of lesion

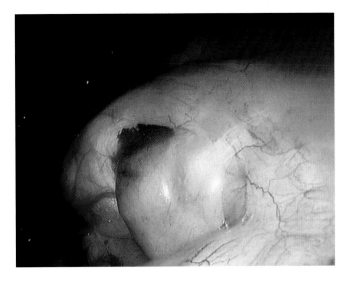

Figure 10.2 Methylene blue injected at the site of the lesion

Port positions

The position of the ports for laparoscopic colectomy depends on the nature and the site of the operation

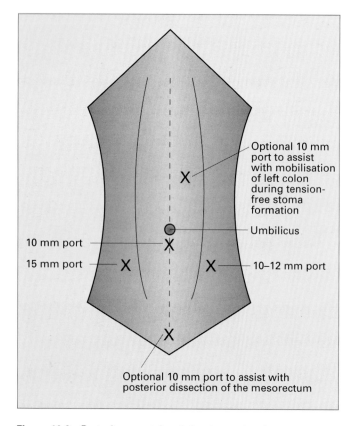

Figure 10.3 Port placement for abdomino-perineal resection

Optional 10 mm port to assist with mobilisation of left colon during tension-free stoma formation

Umbilicus

10 mm port

15 mm port

10–12 mm port

Optional 10 mm port to assist with posterior dissection of the mesorectum

(Figure 10.3). The surgeon stands opposite the side of the planned resection. It is sensible to start with a limited number of ports and to introduce others as the operation progresses: this allows later ports to be sited more appropriately. It is important to try to position the main working ports at 90° to each other and to avoid placing them too close together. For pelvic procedures, the surgeon should err on the side of siting the cannulas too low, because the instruments may not be long enough to complete the procedure easily. If intracorporeal division of structures is anticipated, at least one 12 mm port is required for the endoscopically placed stapling device (a 15 mm port is necessary if the Multifire Endo-GIA instrument is used).

Patient position

For operations on the pelvis the patient is placed in a steep Trendelenburg position to reduce the small bowel into the upper abdomen. Similarly, adjusting the patient's position on the table to head up and lateral tilt will help during mobilisation of the hepatic and splenic flexures. After careful observation of the abdominal contents, particularly the liver, the colon is mobilised with electrocautery scissors using a combination of diathermy, blunt and sharp dissection. Countertraction is achieved by grasping the colon with atraumatic endoscopic forceps. Extreme care must be taken because even these specially designed instruments can tear the bowel if it is handled roughly. During laparoscopic anterior and abdominoperineal resection, further countertraction during the posterior rectal dissection can be accomplished by manipulating an intrarectal metal sizer or a rigid sigmoidoscope. Anterior dissection can be facilitated by introducing a similar instrument into the vagina.

Dissection

Lines of dissection closely follow those of a conventional open procedure. The ureter must be seen clearly during dissection of the sigmoid colon or caecum (Figure 10.4) and is pushed laterally. With good anterior traction on the rectum, excellent views of the splanchnic nerves, the leaves of the mesorectum, and the bloodless "holy plane" can be obtained. Medium sized vessels encountered in the lateral ligaments or at the flexures should be clipped if they are too large for diathermy coagulation.

Resection

Once the relevant portion of the bowel is fully mobilised it can be brought to the surface through a small transverse incision. Alternatively, the bowel and mesenteric vascular supply can be divided intracorporeally using a linear stapler cutter, such as the Endo-GIA, loaded with a haemostatic vascular cartridge (Figure 10.5). Although expensive, this method has the advantage of permitting a more extensive excision of the

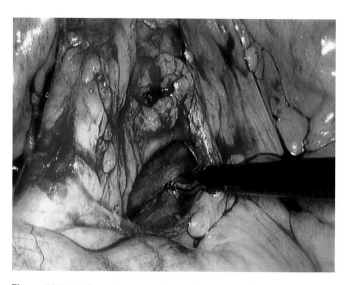

Figure 10.4 Left ureter, seen through an avascular mesenteric window beneath the inferior mesenteric vessels

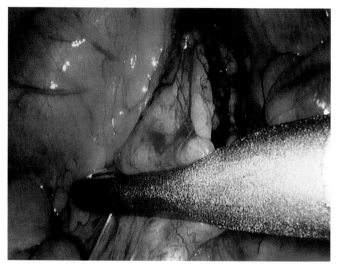

Figure 10.5 Laparoscopic linear stapler cutter dividing the inferior mesenteric vessels

mesentery, which does not need to be dragged out through a small incision before the vessels are divided. Curved or roticulating instruments are particularly helpful in isolating major vessels between avascular mesenteric "windows". Stapling devices may also be used to divide the colon intracorporeally.

Anastomosis and specimen retrieval

Because an incision is usually needed to retrieve the specimen, many surgeons prefer to anastomose the bowel outside the abdominal cavity. Intracorporeal anastomoses are feasible, but until an acceptable method of specimen retrieval is discovered, the extra time and effort needed hardly seems worth while. In malignant disease it is particularly important to ensure that the specimen is not forced through too small an incision; reports of tumour seeding in such wounds have already appeared,[4][5] although this problem might be minimised by irrigating the wound with cancericidal solutions before closure. A completely intracorporeal operation has been described,[6] with removal of the specimen through the open rectal stump but this method still carries a risk of implantation of malignant cells, in addition to damage to the rectum and anal sphincters. Abdomino-perineal resection specimens are removed via the perineal wound in a conventional fashion.

Conclusion

There is certainly a place for laparoscopically assisted colorectal surgery, but it should not be widely introduced until techniques have been evaluated in specialist centres. A recent report suggests that there is no definite cost-benefit in these patients, unlike laparoscopic cholecystectomy.[4] This is largely due to the fact that patients who have undergone laparoscopic procedures that need to be converted to open surgery combine increased operating costs with a traditionally prolonged hospital stay. However, in carefully selected patients the laparoscopic approach has potential advantages. This type of surgery is demanding on the operator and, particularly, the assistants; it should be undertaken only in optimal circumstances.

1 Wexner SD, Cohen SM, Johansen OB, Noguera JJ, Jagelman DC. Laparoscopic colorectal surgery: a prospective assessment and current perspective. *Br J Surg* 1993;**80**:1602–5.
2 Falk PM, Beart Jr RW, Wexner JD *et al.* Laparoscopic colectomy: a critical appraisal. *Dis Colon Rectum* 1993;**36**:28–34.
3 O'Rourke NA, Heald RJ. Laparoscopic surgery for colorectal cancer. *Br J Surg* 1993;**80**:1229–30.
4 Nduka LC, Monson JRT, Menzies-Gow N, Darzi A. Abdominal wall metastases following laparoscopy. *Br J Surg* 1994;**81**:648–52.
5 Fusco MA, Paluzzi MW. Abdominal wall recurrence after laparoscopic-assisted colectomy for adenocarcinoma of the colon. Report of a case. *Dis Colon Rectum* 1993;**36**:858–61.
6 Phillips EH, Franklin M, Carroll BJ, Fallas MJ, Ramos R, Rosenthal D. Laparoscopic colectomy. *Ann Surg* 1992;**216**:703–7.

11 Laparoscopic surgery in gynaecology

A R B Smith

Laparoscopy has been widely used by gynaecologists over the past three decades for diagnostic purposes (Figure 11.1).

- Diagnosis of pain and infertility
- Surgery to the uterine adnexa and environs
- Surgery to the uterus
- Surgery for pelvic visceral prolapse

More recently, therapeutic procedures have been performed laparoscopically. To prevent these techniques falling into disrepute surgeons must be properly trained and the procedures assessed thoroughly.

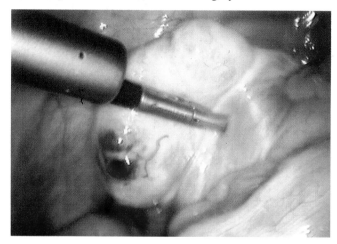

Figure 11.1 Diagnostic laparoscopy showing corpus luteal cyst in left ovary

Diagnosis of pain and infertility

Determining the cause of pelvic pain, both acute and chronic, is a common problem for gynaecologists.

Ectopic pregnancy

- Unhelpful or misleading history
- Patient unaware of pregnancy
- Pain attributed to recurrent pelvic inflammatory disease
- Pain minimal or absent, even with haemoperitoneum
- Massive blood loss without evident shock

This is a potentially life threatening cause of acute pelvic pain, although the widespread use of laparoscopy is reducing the mortality rates.[1] It may be a difficult problem to diagnose and a number of investigations are used to aid in making the diagnosis, including measurements of serum and urinary human chorionic gonadotrophin (HCG) levels, ultrasound scanning and laparoscopy. Increased sensitivity and specificity of HCG assays and the improved resolution of ultrasound scanning have reduced the number of negative laparoscopies when ectopic pregnancy is suspected. However, laparoscopy still provides the definitive diagnosis in most cases,[2,3] enables location of the ectopic, and allows assessment of the degree of haemoperitoneum (Figure 11.2).

Laparoscopic surgery to uterine adnexa:
- Ectopic pregnancy
- Endometriosis
- Ovarian cysts
- Ovarian entrapment
- Irritable bowel syndrome
- Infertility

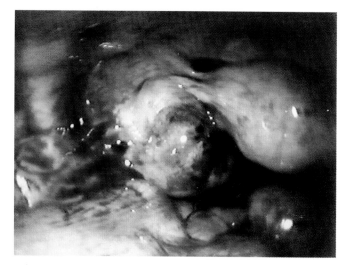

Figure 11.2 View into pelvis, showing left ectopic pregnancy

Endometriosis

This may appear as small red, white or black spots (Figure 11.3), depending on whether the disease is active, inactive or contains old blood. The common sites

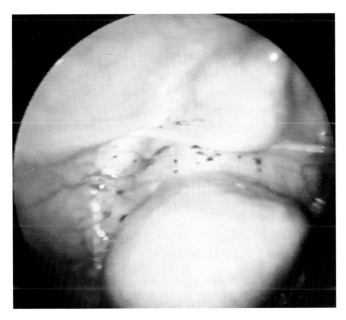

Figure 11.3 Black spots of endometriosis, anterior to uterus

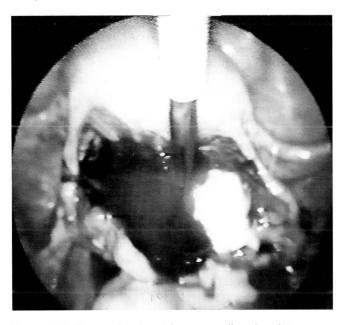

Figure 11.5 Ruptured endometrioma, revealing chocolate coloured contents

for endometriosis are the pouch of Douglas, around the uterosacral ligaments, on the side wall of the pelvis, and on the ovary. It may present as a large cyst (endometrioma), seen in Figure 11.4 lying posterior to the uterus, and often contains chocolate coloured fluid (Figure 11.5). Endometriosis may produce extensive scarring and adhesions, which are generally more dense than those following infection, making adhesiolysis more difficult.

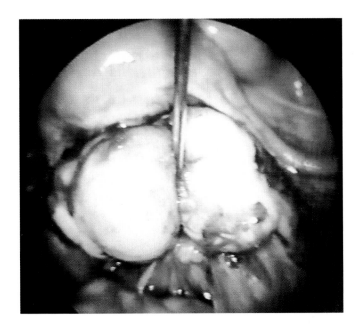

Figure 11.4 Endometrioma in the pouch of Douglas

Ovarian cysts

These may rupture, become torted, or undergo haemorrhage into the cyst. Cysts are often detected by ultrasonography, but whether they cause the abdominal pain is usually determined only at laparoscopy. The fallopian tubes may also become torted, which may cause pelvic pain (Figure 11.6).

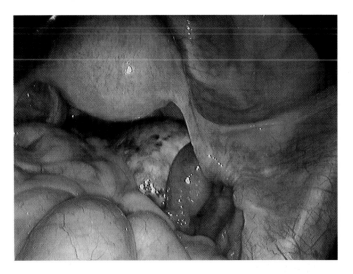

Figure 11.6 View of pelvis showing torsion of right fallopian tube

Pelvic inflammatory disease

This continues to be a common problem, especially in young women. Acutely the fallopian tubes are oedematous with increased vascularity, and there may be an exudate in the pouch of Douglas. A pyosalpinx is diagnosed by tubal swelling or pus draining from the tubes, but in the chronic situation the tubes become occluded and the fimbrial ends clubbed. A hydrosalpinx (a distended tube filled with serous fluid) may form and there may be widespread pelvic adhesions.

Ovarian entrapment

This is usually due to adhesions following hysterectomy, but may also be secondary to pelvic infection or endometriosis. The ovary tends to adhere to the side wall of the pelvis, and care must be taken to avoid ureteric injury when releasing it surgically.

Mid cycle ovulation pain may present as a gynaecological emergency. Although many women are aware of such pain on a regular basis it may present as a one off episode mimicking ectopic pregnancy.

Irritable bowel syndrome

This is a very common complaint in young women and the symptoms may be cyclical, causing it to be confused with a gynaecological disorder. In such situations the diagnosis must be made only after excluding gynaecological and other gastrointestinal causes for the pain.

Infertility

Diagnostic laparoscopy is an important tool in the investigation of infertility, to detect pathology (pelvic inflammatory disease, endometriosis) and to check tubal patency and ovarian function. Tubal patency is demonstrated by injecting methylene blue through the uterine cervix and observing its flow along the fallopian tubes and through the fimbrial ends. Patency may also be demonstrated by hysterosalpingogram, but a laparoscopy allows the pelvic anatomy to be visualised directly. The ovaries can also be inspected for evidence of ovulation (presence of a follicle or corpus luteum).

Surgery to the uterine adnexa and environs

Sterilisation

Laparoscopic surgery has been employed for many years to perform female sterilisation. This has been achieved by applying an occlusive clip (Figure 11.7) (for example Filshie clip, Hulka clip, Falope ring) across the fallopian tubes or using diathermy to burn, and thus occlude, the tubes. An additional port allows more extensive surgery to be performed on the fallopian tubes and ovaries.

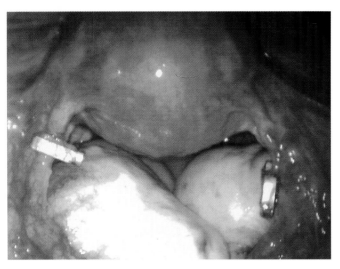

Figure 11.7 Clips on fallopian tubes (placed some time previously). Note the right sided clip is dislodged.

Salpingectomy or salpingotomy

Salpingectomy or salpingotomy for ectopic pregnancy is one of the most useful applications of gynaecological laparoscopic surgery. If the fallopian tube has been ruptured or is greatly distorted by the pregnancy, salpingectomy is advisable. If the fallopian tube has not ruptured, and the swelling is less than 3 cm in diameter, the tube may be opened on the antimesenteric border, the pregnancy aspirated, haemostasis secured, and the tube left unclosed (Figure 11.8). The patient is then monitored by serial measurements of HCG levels to ensure that all the placental tissue has been removed. Laparoscopy may also be used to inject the ectopic pregnancy with methotrexate or dextrose solution, with similar follow up to ensure complete removal of placental tissue. Laparoscopic salpingectomy and other tubal surgery in experienced hands offers real advantages to the patient over open surgery.

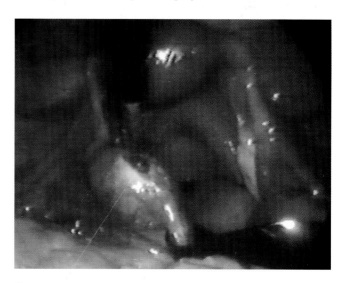

Figure 11.8 View into pelvis showing an ectopic pregnancy and fallopian tube being opened

Pelvic adhesiolysis

Pelvic adhesions following infection, endometriosis or previous surgery are a common cause of morbidity, especially pain and infertility. Adhesiolysis at laparotomy is often followed by the formation of further adhesions, whereas laparoscopic adhesiolysis may be performed using diathermy (monopolar or bipolar) or laser and may reduce the risk of subsequent adhesion formation.

Endometriosis

Endometriosis may be treated laparoscopically, but whether surgery is better than medical therapy for mild endometriosis has not been established. In severe disease, for example when there are ovarian endometriotic cysts, a laparoscopic approach by an experienced surgeon may achieve adequate treatment and avoid the need for laparotomy.

Ovarian laparoscopic surgery

Ovarian laparoscopic surgery (Figure 11.9) is controversial as there is a risk of malignancy in an ovarian cyst, even in young women, and spillage of a cyst's contents during surgery may worsen the prognosis. Reports of metastases in the laparoscopic port wounds indicate that implantation may occur unless care is taken when removing the specimen. Spillage may be prevented by performing ovarian cystectomy within a transparent impermeable bag within the pelvis, but this requires additional skills. The specimen may be removed, still held in the impermeable bag, either through an enlarged port hole or through the posterior vaginal fornix. Treatment of polycystic ovarian syndrome (oligomenorrhoea, hirsutism, infertility) by multiple drilling of the ovaries has been applied successfully in some women. However, this procedure carries the risk of adhesion formation, which may adversely affect fertility.

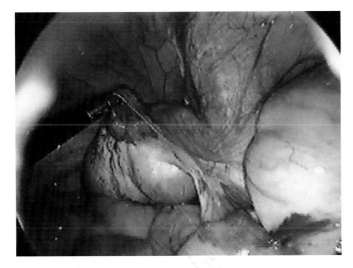

Figure 11.9 Left: ovarian cyst lying alongside bowel

Hazards

The main hazard of surgery to the uterine adnexa is injury to the ureter or major pelvic vessels caused by adhesions to the pelvic side wall. To avoid this hazard an extraperitoneal dissection may be required. Surgery of the ovary in the presence of adhesions to the wall of the pelvis should be performed only by an experienced laparoscopic surgeon.

Conservative uterine surgery

Uterine fibroids (myomas) may produce heavy periods, subfertility and pelvic pain. Submucosal fibroids distort the endometrial cavity and interfere with menstruation and fertility. They may lie deep within the myometrium and so their removal can be difficult and vascular. The morbidity from haemorrhage is greater with myomectomy than with hysterectomy, and laparoscopic myomectomy has only a limited role at present.

Laparoscopic hysterectomy

This may be subtotal (leaving the cervix in situ) or total. The advantages with the former method are that it is not essential to open the vagina, and that preservation of the cervix reduces the risk of damaging the ureters which lie lateral to the cervix before entering the bladder. There is currently debate as to whether the cervix is important for normal sexual function; the protagonists of subtotal hysterectomy cite that cervical preservation is preferable for this reason. The disadvantages of subtotal hysterectomy include the risk of malignant change in the cervix, and if any endometrium remains then cyclical bleeding may occur. Currently 85% of hysterectomies in the UK are performed abdominally, suggesting the need for training in laparoscopic and vaginal hysterectomy. The first laparoscopic hysterectomy was reported by Reich in 1989,[4] and large series have been reported since.

Total hysterectomy

Position

The patient is placed in the flattened lithotomy position, the bladder is emptied, and the abdomen is insufflated with CO_2 in the routine manner. The laparoscope is inserted via the umbilical port. Additional ports are placed lateral to the inferior epigastric artery (Figure 11.10). The uterus is cannulated so that it can be manipulated from below to aid intra-abdominal surgery.

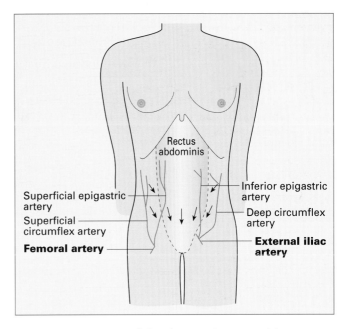

Figure 11.10 Diagram of sites for port placements (↓)

The top pedicle

The top pedicle is approached first, surgery here involving ligating the ovarian ligament, the fallopian tube, the round ligament, and the tubal artery. The vascular pedicle may be dealt with using bipolar diathermy, a multiple stapling device, or a ligature. The multiple stapling device seems to be the most popular at present, although it is also the most expensive. If the ovaries are to be removed the ovarian vessels within the infundibular ligament must be ligated, a manoeuvre that is easily performed using the multiple stapling device. Once the top pedicle has been removed the bladder is reflected from the cervix to give clear access to the uterine artery pedicle. Some surgeons prefer to secure this pedicle vaginally (laparoscopically assisted hysterectomy) when the bladder is also reflected from below. Figure 11.11 shows the view of the uterus after the anterior peritoneum has been elevated and the right ovary and pedicle separated.

Ureteric injury

With reflection of the bladder from the cervix the vagina is visible and the uterine artery pedicle may be secured by diathermy or stapling. Some surgeons advocate skeletalisation of the uterine vessels before clipping them individually. At this stage care must be taken not to injure the ureter, which runs 1–2 cm lateral to the cervix. Ureteric stents may be used at this stage to help protect the ureter. Using the multiple stapling device the pedicle is secured more laterally than would be the case at open operation, which puts the ureter more at risk. The advantage of using ureteric stents is that they can not be moved if the stapling device is closed over them, therefore the ability to move the stent can be checked before the stapling device is fired and the device opened and repositioned before firing if necessary. Transilluminated stents have been used, but they are not visible through the laparoscope at the point where the ureter is most at risk.

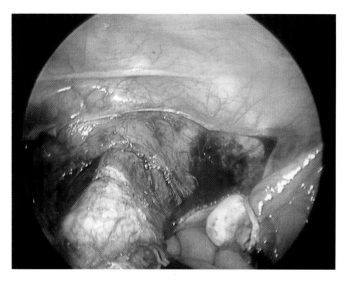

(a)

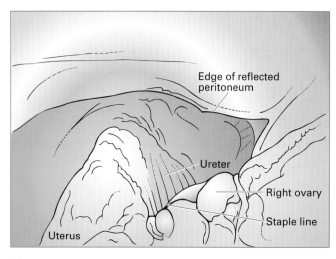

(b)

Figure 11.11 Laparoscopic hysterectomy—right ovary and pedicle separated from uterus

Vaginal aspects of surgery

After the uterine artery pedicle is divided the surgeon may perform the rest of the procedure vaginally, or may partially divide the uterosacral ligaments laparoscopically (by diathermy and scissors) and open the vagina laparoscopically. These last two steps make the vaginal part of the procedure easier to perform. Vaginally the cervix is circumscribed and the uterosacral ligaments ligated, the uterus is removed and the vagina closed with interrupted or continuous sutures. Metal staples could injure the woman's partner during intercourse, and so should not be used to close the vagina.

Subtotal hysterectomy

The top pedicles are secured as described for total hysterectomy. The uterus is then transected at the level

of the internal cervical os, and morcellated so that it may be removed. The disadvantage of this technique is that histological examination is much more difficult with a specimen of many pieces than with a single specimen. If the specimen needs to be kept intact it may be removed via an incision in the posterior fornix.

Complications

Wound haematoma

Wound haematoma and other complications of laparoscopic procedures may occur. The inferior epigastric vessels are particularly vulnerable when siting the lateral ports.

Ureteric injury

Ureteric injury may occur on the side wall of the pelvis when securing the ovarian pedicle or close to the cervix when the uterine artery pedicle is being secured.

Bladder injury

The bladder may be injured during hysterectomy, especially after previous caesarean section when the bladder is often adherent to the cervix.

Pelvic haematoma

The incidence of pelvic haematoma should be lower with laparoscopic hysterectomy than open procedures, as the pedicles are all visible via the laparoscope at the end of the procedure. However, haematomas still occur and it may be necessary to observe the pedicles after releasing the pneumoperitoneum, so that the tamponade effect of the high pressure is removed. Secondary haemorrhage may occur, as with any hysterectomy, and this tends to present with vaginal bleeding approximately 10 days after surgery.

Benefits

Postoperative recovery appears to be improved with laparoscopic surgery. Most women stay in hospital for 48 h after surgery and are fit to return to normal activities within 3–4 weeks.

Laparoscopic surgery for prolapse

- Colposuspension
- Uterine malposition
- Uterine prolapse
- Vault prolapse and enterocoele

Laparoscopic colposuspension

Anterior vaginal wall prolapse is often accompanied by stress incontinence. Laparoscopic colposuspension was first reported in 1993 by Liu,[5] and it is still too early to be able to make valid comparisons with results of standard techniques (at least 2 years is required). It does appear that bladder neck elevation comparable to open colposuspension can be achieved, with a considerable reduction in operative and postoperative morbidity. The retropubic space may be entered directly or via the peritoneal cavity, and the space is opened by blunt dissection and CO_2 insufflation because it normally contains filmy connective tissue. The bladder may be mobilised from the paraurethral fascia in the conventional manner and sutures placed to approximate the paraurethral fascia and Cooper's ligament (Figure 11.12). If the patient is able to void following surgery then hospitalisation is required only for 48 h. In the USA patients may be discharged after 24 h with a suprapubic catheter in place, returning for assessment after 7 days to discover if voiding is possible. Voiding problems are the main complication of this type of surgery.

Surgery for uterine malposition

Laparoscopic ventrosuspension to correct retroversion may be of value when performed in conjunction with laparoscopic adhesiolysis. If the uterus is fixed by

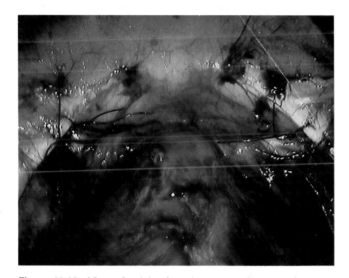

Figure 11.12 View of pelvis after placement of sutures for colposuspension

adhesions in the retroverted position anteversion of the uterus may prevent reformation of the adhesions. Ventrosuspension can be performed via the laparoscope by suture plication of the round ligaments.

Laparoscopic surgery for uterine prolapse

Conventional conservative surgery for uterine prolapse includes a Manchester repair (anterior vaginal repair, amputation of cervix, shortening of uterosacral ligaments, and posterior vaginal repair). It is possible to reduce the uterine prolapse laparoscopically by shortening and approximating the uterosacral ligaments. This reduces the risk of enterocoele and requires no more than 24 h in hospital. The long term benefits of this procedure are not yet known.

Vault prolapse and enterocoele

Prolapse of the vaginal vault and enterocoele are not uncommon sequelae to hysterectomy. If the uterosacral ligaments are still present a vaginal repair may be performed satisfactorily, but commonly these ligaments are in poor condition. Sacrocolpopexy has been advocated for supporting the vaginal vault by fixing a prolene mesh from the top of the vagina to the sacrum. This may be performed laparoscopically, suturing the mesh to the vaginal vault and then stapling it to the periosteum of the sacrum. Additional support may be obtained by securing the mesh to the posterior vaginal wall as well as to the vault.

1 Zorn JR, Risquez F, Cedard L. Ectopic pregnancy. *Curr Opin Obstet Gynecol* 1992;4:238–45.
2 Lundorff P. Modern management of ectopic pregnancy. Early recognition, laparoscopic treatment and fertility prospects. *Acta Obstet Gynecol Scand* 1992;71:158–9.
3 Achiran R *et al.* Pelvic sonography and serum beta HCG versus diagnostic laparoscopy in the diagnosis of stable patients suspected as ectopic pregnancy. *Clin Exp Obstet Gynecol* 1992;166:1062–71.
4 Riech H, De Caprior J, McGlynn F. Laparoscopic hysterectomy. *J Gynecol Surg* 1989;5:213–16.
5 Liu CY. Laparoscopic retropubic colposuspension (Burch procedure)—a review of 58 cases. *J Reprod Med* 1993;38:526–30.

12 Laparoscopic surgery in urology

Mark S Cade, Adrian D Joyce

Urologists have used minimally invasive techniques for many years, and most operative urology is carried out endoscopically. Transurethral prostatectomy remains the archetypal minimally invasive procedure and most bladder tumours are managed cystoscopically. More recently, ureteroscopy has made visualisation of the ureters possible and ureteroscopic stone surgery is available in most large urological centres. Percutaneous nephrolithotomy was introduced in the early 1980s and is now widely available. Its use, and that of extracorporeal shockwave lithotripsy have made open renal stone surgery a rare occurrence.

In spite of the widespread use of operative endoscopy, urologists were slow to adopt operative laparoscopy. This is now being corrected and the urologists' endoscopic skills are being applied in the abdominal cavity as well as in the urinary tract.[1]

The role of laparoscopy in urology

- Diagnosis, for example intra-abdominal testicle
- Simple operative techniques such as ligation of varicocoele, mobilisation of intra-abdominal testicle
- Solid organ resection, for example nephrectomy, lymph node dissection
- Complex reconstructive surgery, for example ileal conduit urinary diversion, pyeloplasty

The first three uses of laparoscopy are currently practised; the fourth is being developed, but is at present limited to a few centres. A major problem is the restriction imposed by current technology, but if the present pace of technological advance continues the difficulties of access to the pelvis and retroperitoneum will soon be overcome and more complex operative urology will become widespread.

Diagnostic procedures

Non-palpable testis

The non-palpable testicle is most reliably identified by laparoscopy, although it is sometimes necessary to divide

adhesions to the sigmoid colon in order to identify the left testicle. The testicular vessels may be seen and traced to an intra-abdominal testicle or to the deep inguinal ring. The testicle, once identified, can be biopsied or the testicular vessels divided between pairs of clips and the testicle can be mobilised and removed or, if appropriate, left in position as the first stage of a Fowler–Stephens orchidopexy.[2] The second stage may be performed as an open procedure approximately 6 weeks later. In the adult primary removal of an intra-abdominal testis is advocated.

Simple operative urology

Varicocoele

A varicocoele is an abnormal tortuosity and dilatation of the testicular veins within the spermatic cord, occurring predominantly on the left side and probably related to the difference between the venous drainage of the two sides. Varicocoeles can cause subfertility or a dragging sensation in the affected testicle.

Open varicocoele surgery involves a retroperitoneal, scrotal or inguinal approach. Recurrence is a problem even for the experienced surgeon; the rate is 5–45% following surgery, although recurrence of discomfort is unusual. The best results have been obtained by an open microsurgical technique in which the gubernacular vessels are divided, and the lymphatics and testicular arteries preserved.[3]

Laparoscopic varicocoelectomy

Laparoscopic varicocoelectomy is a direct application of the technique of open high ligation of the testicular vein. The magnification afforded by the laparoscope has allowed advances in this technique as all the vessels may be seen and differentiated using the Doppler ultrasound probe. Thus, the testicular artery and lymphatics may be left in place while ligating the abnormal veins.

Position

The patient is placed supine with 20–25° head down tilt. As long as the bladder has been emptied no catheter is required. The abdomen is insufflated, a 10 mm port inserted at the umbilicus and two further 10 mm ports placed at the lateral edge of the rectus.

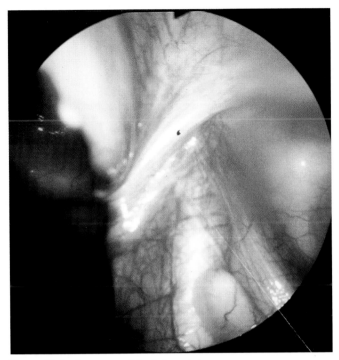

Figure 12.1 Anatomy of the internal ring

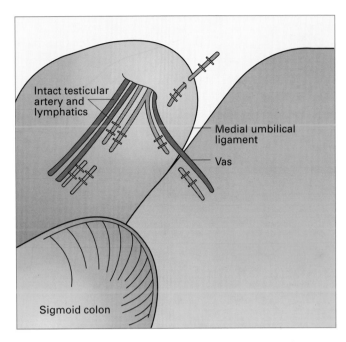

Figure 12.3 Diagrammatic representation of laparoscopic varicocoele ligation

Procedure

The vas is identified where it leaves the internal ring to pass medially and downwards (Figure 12.1), and dissection performed away from the vas. The peritoneum is incised longitudinally for 2 cm just lateral to the testicular vessels, and the incision may be extended transversely across the vessels if necessary. The internal spermatic fascia is opened separately in order to identify the individual veins and their accompanying lymphatics (Figure 12.2). The veins may then be clipped and divided individually, preserving the arteries. The vas is exposed through a separate incision in order to identify any aberrant obturator veins, which can be diathermied or clipped (Figure 12.3) if necessary. At the medial end of the canal a 1 cm incision will identify the external spermatic vein, which should be clipped and divided. After adequate haemostasis has been achieved the ports are removed, the abdomen deflated and the wounds closed.

Solid organ resection

Laparoscopic pelvic lymphadenectomy

The laparoscopic dissection of pelvic lymph nodes is possible, but is justifiable only if subsequent management will be altered by the finding of metastases. Surgical staging of nodes is more accurate than non-invasive staging, but will not remove all relevant nodes and can not be regarded as radical surgical treatment for lymph node positive disease. The extent of the node dissection depends on the lymphatic drainage of the relevant organ: the bladder drains to the external iliac nodes, the prostate to the internal iliac and sacral nodes, the cervix and lower uterus drain laterally via the perimetrium to the external iliac nodes, and the upper uterus drains with the ovarian lymphatics to the para-aortic nodes.

Laparoscopic pelvic lymphadenectomy has a role in staging apparently localised prostatic carcinoma before radical prostatectomy, but the role of lymph node dissection is less well defined for bladder cancer because of the lack of satisfactory treatment for patients with positive nodes: two studies have shown that micrometastases in pelvic nodes make no difference to survival after radical cystectomy.[6] Staging for gynaecological malignancy should help avoid unnecessary radical surgery in patients with unsuspected metastases.

There has been a move to less radical node dissection, urologists concentrating on the nodes in the obturator fossa along the external iliac vein and the hypogastric artery. The cranial and caudal limits of the dissection are the iliac bifurcation and Cloquet's node or Cooper's ligament.

Position

The patient is placed supine with a 20–25° head down tilt. Thromboembolic deterrent stockings should be worn for deep vein thrombosis prophylaxis. Port placement and insufflation are as described for

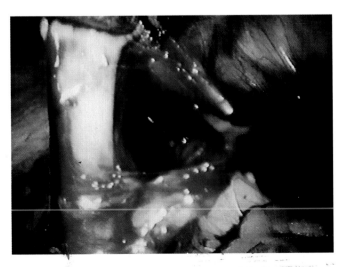

Figure 12.2 Dilated spermatic vessel

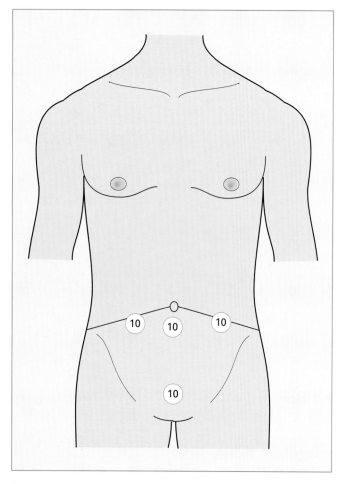

Figure 12.4 Trocar sites for laparoscopic pelvic lymph node dissection

laparoscopic varicocoelectomy, with a fourth port placed in the midline 3–4 cm above the pubic symphysis (Figure 12.4).

Dissection

The landmarks for dissection are the umbilical ligament medially, the pubic bone anteriorly and the external iliac vessels laterally. The peritoneum is incised along the medial border of the external iliac vein and the fibrofatty tissue around the vein cleared. The obturator fossa is dissected and its contents removed to expose the obturator nerve (Figure 12.5). The dissection proceeds

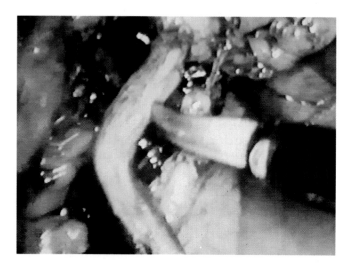

Figure 12.5 Mobilisation of obturator nodal package

lateral to the medial umbilical ligament, with care taken not to damage the ureter where it crosses the ligament. The pieces of tissue are counted as they are removed, placed in the paracolic gutter to be marked according to its side (Figure 12.6), and removed in a retrieval bag at the end of the procedure. Large lymphatic vessels may need to be clipped but smaller ones can be sealed with diathermy. Closure is as described above.

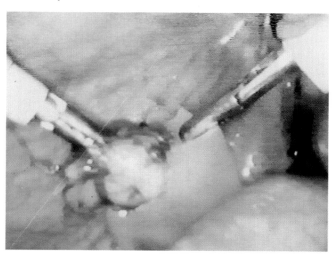

Figure 12.6 Placement of nodes in retrieval bag

Complications

Haemorrhage may lead to the necessity for laparotomy. Other complications include deep vein thrombosis, accidental cystostomy, retroperitoneal abscess, and obturator nerve palsy. The morbidity for these procedures appears to be much lower than that for open lymphadenectomy.

Extraperitoneal pelviscopy

An alternative to the above technique is to insufflate the extraperitoneal space via a suprapubic placement of the Veress needle. Once the space is distended the nodes may be dissected without entering the peritoneal cavity. However, this approach seems to have a higher incidence of lymphocoele, and drainage is required.

Para-aortic lymphadenectomy

The usual reason for the removal of para-aortic nodes is to treat residual nodal masses following chemotherapy for testicular teratoma. The removal of all lymphatic tissue would be very difficult with the equipment currently available and the restricted access to the retroperitoneum, so only significantly enlarged residual tissue is removed. The procedure may be performed transperitoneally or extraperitoneally, but most experience is with the former.[6]

Position

The patient is placed in the lateral position, affected side uppermost, with the table broken between the rib cage and the iliac crest. Urethral, but not ureteric, catheterisation is used. The Veress needle is inserted at the edge of the rectus sheath at the level of the umbilicus. After insufflation the endoscope is inserted via a 10 mm port at the same site and two secondary ports placed in the mid-clavicular line. A 12 mm port is placed at least 2 cm below the ribs to allow freer movement. These two ports are used for the instrumentation.

Dissection

The peritoneal reflection lateral to the colon is divided and the colon mobilised medially with the aid of gravity. It is helpful for the colon to have been emptied using an enema before surgery. The colon is mobilised and a 5 mm port placed in the mid-axillary line for lateral retraction. A 10 mm port is placed in the midline between the xiphisternum and umbilicus so that the fan retractor can hold the colon medially.

The para-aortic dissection begins at the bifurcation and proceeds proximally, clipping or dividing vessels with the Endo-GIA 30 stapler. When dissection is completed the tissue is removed is in extraction bag, and a suction drain placed into the node bed via the 5 mm port. Closure is as described earlier.

Laparoscopic nephrectomy

The high incidence of morbidity with open nephrectomy is a compelling reason for an alternative approach, and the advent of impermeable bags for the retrieval of large volumes of tissue has made laparoscopic nephrectomy feasible. The first such procedure was performed in 1991 by Clayman,[7] and has been applied to both benign and malignant disease. A patient may return home 3–4 days after radical nephrectomy if performed laparoscopically.

Relative contraindications include the possibility of dense adhesions after previous open renal surgery or after perinephric abscess. The presence of renal tumour breaching the capsule or invading the renal vein are absolute contraindications.

Position and dissection

The patient is positioned in the loin position (Figure 12.7) and the Veress needle inserted at the edge of the rectus sheath, at the level of the umbilicus. Four ports are generally used (Figure 12.8).

After mobilisation of the right or left colon (see above) the ureter should be identified as it passes over the iliac vessels (Figure 12.9). This is clipped and divided before being retracted proximally to the kidney. The gonadal vessels are clipped and divided where they cross the ureter. If the kidney is hydronephrotic it should be aspirated at this stage. The perinephric fat is incised and

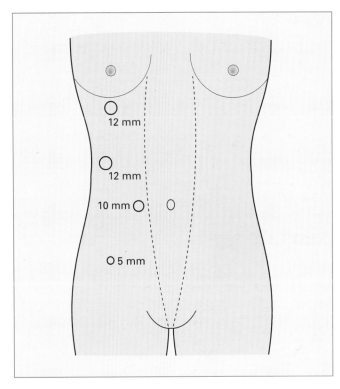

Figure 12.8 Trocar sites for transperitoneal laparoscopic nephrectomy

the renal pedicle displayed by gentle dissection at the hilum while applying lateral traction on the kidney (Figure 12.10). When the vessels are clearly exposed they can be clipped if less than 5 mm diameter; more commonly they are divided separately with the Endo-GIA 30 stapler (Figures 12.11 and 12.12). The freed kidney is placed in an organ retrieval bag and the neck of the bag delivered to the body surface while the kidney bed is inspected and haemostasis is achieved. The kidney is morcellated in the retrieval bag before being removed piecemeal. It may be necessary to enlarge the port to 20 mm to remove all the tissue. The operative

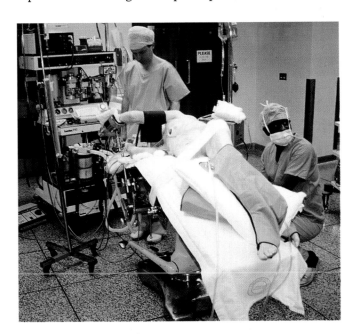

Figure 12.7 Position of patient for laparoscopic nephrectomy

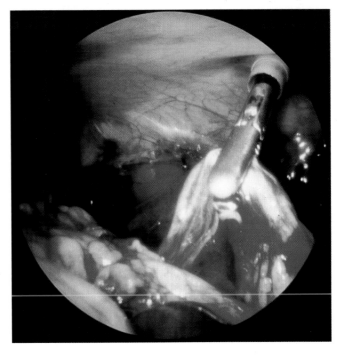

Figure 12.9 Identification of ureter after colonic mobilisation

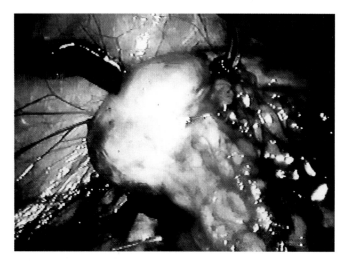

Figure 12.10   Elevation of mobilised kidney (right)

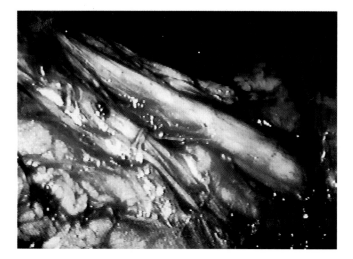

Figure 12.11   Identification of renal artery and vein

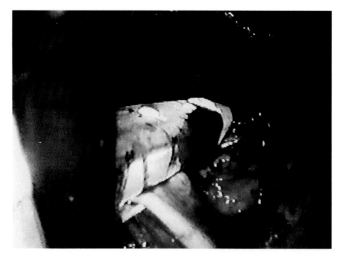

Figure 12.12   Venous haemostasis secured with Endo-GIA stapler

site is drained, usually for 24 hours, the ports removed and the wounds closed.

If a nephroureterectomy is indicated for benign disease a further port is needed at the edge of the rectus sheath in line with the anterior superior iliac spine. Dissection may then be carried out to within 1–2 cm of the bladder and the ureter clipped and divided. If the disease is a renal transitional cell carcinoma the ureteric

orifice can be circumcised transurethrally at the start of the procedure, allowing all the ureter to be removed. An indwelling catheter is required for 10 days after this procedure.

Radical nephrectomy may be performed in a similar fashion, but dissection is carried out around the perinephric fat rather than around the renal capsule. This may be easier than dissecting through the fat of a previously infected kidney.

Complications

In a series of 40 transperitoneal nephrectomies two required conversion to open nephrectomy as they had staghorn calculi and densely adherent kidneys. Postoperative haemorrhage requiring transfusion occurred in three patients, two of whom required laparotomy for the management of this. One patient suffered cardiac dysrhythmias due to persistent metabolic acidosis; this patient's surgery lasted 5·5 h. The mean operating time was 2·5 h and the mean inpatient stay 3 days.

Histology

A morcellated specimen causes obvious problems with histological examination, especially staging in cases of malignancy. Preoperative imaging should be used to stage the tumour.

Laparoscopic colposuspension

Laparoscopic colposuspension has recently been described.[8] The operation involves insufflation of the retropubic space and introduction of the telescope and dissection instruments. The paravaginal tissues may then be directly sutured to the ileopectineal ligament as in the Burch colposuspension. As an alternative, a modified Stamey procedure may be followed, passing the Stamey needle through the retropubic space under direct vision.

Laparoscopic ileal conduit diversion

The performance of laparoscopic cystectomy is possible, but is not presently practicable. A number of patients require urinary diversion for benign disease, many of whom are at high risk after open surgery. The standard procedure is an ileal conduit urinary diversion, which can be performed laparoscopically.[9]

Preparation

A preliminary cystoscopy is performed and bilateral ureteric stents inserted. The patient is then placed in the supine position with a head down tilt of 20–25°. Urethral catheterisation is required. The Veress needle is introduced and the abdomen insufflated, passing the scope via the umbilical port. Further ports are placed as required to obtain access to the ureters and the ileum. The ureters are identified as they enter the pelvis, dissected down to the bladder and freed from their insertion.

Bowel preparation

Using a separate light source placed through the lower midline port for transillumination, a suitably placed loop of small bowel is identified. This loop is suspended from the anterior abdominal wall by sutures placed percutaneously. It is then isolated on its vascular pedicle using the Endo-GIA 30 stapler to produce a 15 cm length of ileum closed at each end. Anastomosis may be carried out inside the abdomen, but it is usually possible to bring the two ends to the surface through one of the larger port incisions and to perform extracorporeal anastomosis.

The ureteroileal anastomosis may also be performed intra-abdominally, but is more conveniently performed on the surface, leaving the stents in situ. After dropping the anastomosis back into the abdomen, the ileal stoma is created in a standard fashion.

Two drains are placed in the pelvis, one directed to each anastomosis. Closure is as described above.

Laparoscopic partial cystectomy

The indications for this procedure are more limited than for total cystectomy. However, some patients with localised, superficial bladder cancer are suitable for this procedure.

Position and ports
The patient is placed in the supine position with a 20–25° head down tilt. A urethral catheter is inserted and a pneumoperitoneum introduced through a position just lateral to the umbilicus in order to avoid a urachal remnant that may be involved with the tumour. The ports are placed as for an ileal conduit diversion, without the lower midline port.

Procedure
After inspecting the abdominal contents the peritoneum over the dome of the bladder is incised and the superior vesical pedicles divided between clips or with the Endo-GIA stapler. Stay sutures are inserted percutaneously and the relevant part of the bladder resected and placed in a retrieval bag. The bladder is repaired with a continuous suture and the pelvis drained before the specimen is removed. The ports are removed and the fascia sutured, then the skin is closed. The urethral catheter is left in place for 3 weeks. Patients make a rapid recovery with few problems. Normal voiding is restored within 4–6 months.

Laparoscopic retroperitoneal surgery

Direct insufflation of CO_2 into the retroperitoneal space has not been satisfactory, because it produces an uneven space with many fibrous septae. The

introduction of a dissecting balloon by Gaur[10] has enabled surgeons to utilise this approach for several procedures.

Once the relevant ureter has been intubated cystoscopically the patient is placed in the lateral position (diseased side uppermost) and the table broken. A Helmstein balloon is inserted into the extraperitoneal space through a gridiron incision in the flank. The balloon is inflated to a pressure below 100 mmHg, maintained at maximum volume for 35 min and then removed. The space produced is entered with a blunt port under direct vision and held in place with a pursestring suture. Secondary ports are inserted as required.

Ureterolysis involves dissection of the whole of the ureter followed by lateral displacement and fixation to the posterior abdominal wall. Ureterolithotomy is performed by opening the ureter with a knife and removing the stone. The ureter is not sutured but a stent is inserted transcystoscopically and a drain placed to the ureterotomy. Nephrectomy is performed in a manner similar to that for transperitoneal nephrectomy but limitations in space make this approach useful only for the small dysplastic kidney. Pyeloplasty is performed as a dismembered technique with intracorporeal anastomosis by continuous sutures. A guidewire is passed through the anastomosis before completion and a stent passed across the suture line.

At the end of surgery the ports are removed and the incisions closed as described earlier.

The major problem with retroperitoneal endoscopy seems to be the lack of space, the operative field appearing very crowded. Perinephric adhesions are a contraindication to retroperitoneal insufflation, but the technique clearly has great potential.

1 Copcoat MJ, Joyce AD. Laparoscopy in urology. Oxford: Blackwell Scientific Publications, 1994.
2 Elder JS. Laparoscopy and Fowler–Stephens orchidopexy in the management of the non-palpable testis. Urol Clin North Am 1989;16:399–411.
3 Goldstein M, Gilbert D, Dicker AP, Dwosk J, Gnecco C. Microsurgical inguinal varicocoelectomy with delivery of the testis: an artery and lymphatic sparing technique. J Urol 1992;148:1808–11.
4 Copcoat MJ, Wickham JEA. Laparoscopy in urology. Min Inv Ther 1992;1: 337–42.
5 Parra R, Adrus C, Boullier JA. Staging laparoscopic pelvic lymph node dissection: comparison of results with open pelvic lymphadenectomy. J Urol 1992;147:875–8.
6 Janetschek G, Reissigi A, Peschel R, Bartsch G. Laparoscopic retroperitoneal lymphadenectomy for testicular tumour: animal studies and first clinical experience. Min Inv Ther 1992;1:68.
7 Clayman R, Kavoussi L, Soper N et al. Laparoscopic nephrectomy: initial case report. J Urol 1991;146:278–82.
8 Liu CY. Laparoscopic retropubic colposuspension (Burch procedure)—a review of 58 cases. J Reprod Med 1993;387:526–30.
9 Kzminski M, Partamian KO. Case report of laparoscopic ileal loop conduit. J Endourol 1992;6:147–50.
10 Gaur DD. Laparoscopic operative retroperitoneoscopy: use of a new device. J Urol 1992;148:1137–9.

13 Video assisted thoracic surgery

Mark T Jones, T L Hooper

Thoracoscopy was first performed by Jacobeus in 1910 when he introduced a cystoscope into the pleural space in order to examine the visceral pleura. Until recently thoracoscopy was a purely diagnostic procedure, limited by only one person being able to view the pleural cavity at any time. The recent advances in video camera technology, combined with the rapid development of percutaneous endoscopic instruments, has greatly broadened the role of thoracoscopy in diagnosis and opened up numerous possibilities for therapy. The accepted name given to this management approach is video assisted thoracic surgery (VATS).

Indications

Definite indications:
- Diagnosis and management of pleural effusions
- Elective closed lung biopsy
- Diagnosis of indeterminate solitary pulmonary nodule
- Sympathectomy
- Recurrent pneumothorax (especially in the young)
- Pericardial biopsy, window for effusion

Possible indications:
- Malignant pleural effusion
- Empyema
- First time pneumothorax
- Mobilisation of the oesophagus

Indications depending on long term outcome:
- Oesophageal motility disorders
- Antireflux procedures
- Resection of lung cancer
- Thymectomy for myasthenia gravis

Although VATS has been developed only since about 1992, it has been adopted by thoracic surgeons with great enthusiasm, reflected in the rapid and widespread application of this approach to almost all major intrathoracic procedures. However, enthusiasm must be tempered with caution. A clear role for VATS is emerging in the management of certain conditions (such as recurrent pneumothorax) but in other situations, such as the surgery of benign oesophageal disease or resection for malignant pulmonary disease, its role will not emerge until the results can be compared with the current "gold standard".

Absolute contraindications to VATS are the presence of widespread dense pleural adhesions and the inability to tolerate one lung anaesthesia.

Operative set up for VATS

All procedures are carried out under general anaesthesia with a double lumen endotracheal tube and arterial monitoring by pulse oximetry or direct cannulation. The patient is placed in the lateral position for all procedures and should be fully prepared for open thoracotomy if necessary. Mechanical ventilation of the ipsilateral lung is discontinued as soon as satisfactory endotracheal tube placement is confirmed. This enables some degree of resorption atelectasis of the lung to take place while the patient is being prepared and draped. A partial pneumothorax may be induced by the insufflation of air into the pleural space using an 18-gauge needle and syringe, ensuring that the lung collapses away from the port site. Depending on the type of operation usually three stab incisions 15–35 mm in length are necessary (Figure 13.1). Insufflation with CO_2, as used for laparoscopic procedures, is unnecessary and has the associated risk of haemodynamic upset secondary to mediastinal shift. Airtight trocars for sealing the gas within the hemithorax are similarly unnecessary, so screw thread trocars, or "thoracoports", are used, the thread securing the trocar in the soft tissues. The diameters of these trocars will vary according to need and provide a clear channel into the pleural space enabling easy introduction and removal of instruments.

The first incision is made in the sixth or seventh intercostal space in the mid-axillary line, a 10 mm thoracoport is inserted and a 10 mm, 0° rigid telescope and camera attached to a video monitor introduced. The application of an anti-fogging agent and warming the shaft of the telescope with hot saline solution both help to prevent the telescopic lens misting in the chest. The view within the hemithorax is excellent and a careful inspection should be undertaken to identify pathology and to observe appropriate sites for further port placement (Figure 13.2). Additional incisions are usually made one interspace higher in the anterior and posterior

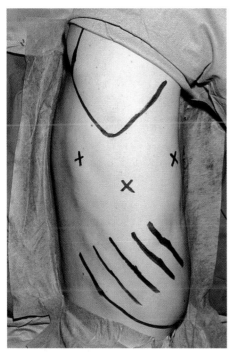

Figure 13.1 Patient in thoracotomy position, port placement

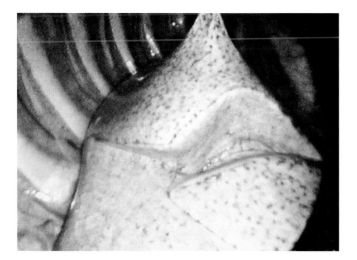

Figure 13.2 View inside right hemithorax. An adhesion is evident

axillary lines. Thoracoports are placed according to need for insertion and manipulation of instruments. If an endoscopic stapling device is to be used a 12 mm port is necessary.

A vast array of instruments is available (Figures 13.3 and 13.4) for most procedures, including extensible

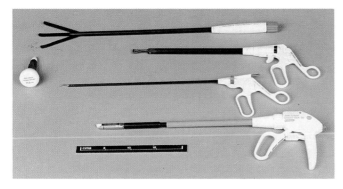

Figure 13.3 Basic set of VATS instruments

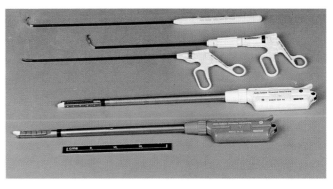

Figure 13.4 Additional instruments commonly used

"fan" retractors of the lung, instruments with "memory" metal for oesophageal retraction, roticulating instruments, and larger capacity endoscopic staplers. Many standard thoracic surgical instruments have been adapted for thorascopic use. Most units will use a mixture of disposable and reusable instruments. A typical operating room scene is as shown in Figure 13.5.

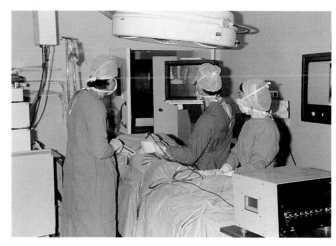

Figure 13.5 Operating room scene

Operative procedures

The instrumentation and camera are arranged to achieve a "triangle of approach" to the target lesion (Figure 13.6). Visualisation of intrathoracic structures is superb, and with appropriate case selection it is possible to undertake most major thoracic operations as VATS procedures.

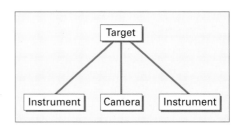

Figure 13.6 Triangle of approach to target lesion in VATS

In the case of pulmonary resection a "utility incision" 5–6 cm long is made in the fifth anterior interspace to enable removal of the specimen. When undertaking the wide variety of therapeutic VATS procedures, different configurations of port placement are required. Two

examples are shown in Figures 13.7 and 13.8, the
camera usually being placed lowermost. It is often
necessary to move the camera and instruments between
ports to optimise the surgical approach.

The key to success is a well planned operation, using
a methodical approach, with careful positioning of the
trocars. Procedures will become quicker and more
straightforward as the surgeon and operating team
acquire experience. Upon completion of the procedure
the chest is irrigated with saline solution and a chest
drain inserted (Figure 13.9).

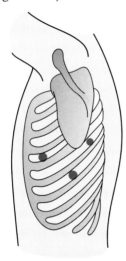

Figure 13.7 Port placement for apical bullous lung disease

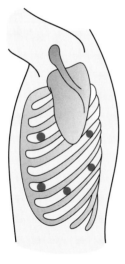

Figure 13.8 Port placement for approach to the distal
oesophagus

Complications

The complications of VATS can be considered as
twofold: complications common to any thoracic
operation and those related specifically to VATS.

Complications common to any thoracic operation

- Wound infection
- Postoperative bleeding
- Arrhythmia
- Prolonged air leak
- Intercostal neuralgia
- Respiratory insufficiency
- Death

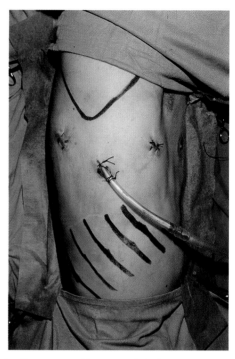

Figure 13.9 Placement of intercostal drain

Most of these complications are reduced in frequency
with VATS, except for air leak, which is prolonged in the
experience of some series. This may be due to
unrecognised trocar or instrumental lung injury,
difficulty in stapler application, lack of expertise in
endoscopic suturing techniques, or possibly accepting
more patients with bullous lung disease for VATS
surgery. Intercostal neuralgia is not uncommon after
open thoracic procedures; in VATS this can be lessened
by correct port placement and avoiding leverage of
instruments or ports. The use of narrower chest drains
and their prompt removal after surgery, combined with
intercostal nerve block and the use of non-steroidal anti-
inflammatory drugs, is also beneficial.

Complications specific to VATS

- Uncontrolled bleeding
- Haemodynamic compromise
- Compromise of the procedure
- Tumour seeding of the chest wall
- Inability to locate solitary pulmonary
  nodules
- Incomplete tumour staging

At all times the surgeon must be prepared to convert
the procedure to an open operation. The excellent
visualisation afforded by VATS should result in few
instances of major haemorrhage. Any suspicion that the
management of the patient is being compromised by this
minimally invasive approach must be followed by open
thoracotomy. Malignant tissue should be brought
through the chest wall only after it has been enclosed in
a protective bag, the only exception being a tumour
deeply placed in lung tissue. Useful aids to the precise
localisation of pulmonary nodules include careful
correlation of the site of the mass to its position on
computed tomography, achievement of full lung

collapse, careful palpation of the lung, needle localisation, and intraoperative ultrasound.

Specific pitfalls and hazards of VATS

- Increased expense
- Prolonged operation time
- Overextension of indications
- Overextension of operability
- Ignorance of one's place on the learning curve

Many of these appear to have an adverse effect on current practice. Economic considerations figure strongly in the uptake of this new surgical approach. It is especially important that VATS is seen to be safe, that the results achieved are no worse than with current approaches, and that it confers a benefit to the patient.

Benefits

Patients undergoing VATS experience less postoperative pain, and stay in hospital for shorter periods on average than those undergoing open procedures. Patients are able to return to normal activities earlier than after open techniques, and the cosmetic appearances of three stab incisions in Langer's lines is superior.

For the ideal indications shown, the shorter time in the operating room and shorter hospital stay should translate into a cost saving to offset the increased cost of instrumentation.

14 Minimal access ENT surgery

Timothy J Rockley

Otolaryngology has developed rapidly in the latter half of the twentieth century, largely due to technological advances that have allowed surgeons to perform operations of increasing complexity. As more sophisticated instruments become available, surgery to the upper respiratory tract and skull base has become less invasive.

Minimal access surgery of the ear, nose, and throat

The development of the operating microscope in the 1950s and 1960s heralded the modern era of surgical otology and laryngology. With the microscope, ear surgeons had a tool that enabled them to devise reliable operations for middle ear reconstruction in the treatment of chronic suppurative otitis media and otosclerosis. Modern ear surgery has always been "minimal access": operations on the middle ear are performed via the ear canal (permeatal approach) or through inconspicuous incisions extending anterosuperiorly from the ear canal (endaural) or behind the ear (postaural). The surgery within the middle ear is performed using fine instruments or microdrills while viewing the operative field through the microscope.

In laryngology, the same operating microscopes were used in conjunction with rigid endoscopes, allowing precise surgical manipulation of the delicate vocal folds under magnification. The practice of endolaryngeal microsurgery has become widespread in the treatment of vocal nodules, laryngeal polyps, leukoplakia (figure 14.1) and small tumours. The development of the surgical laser, delivered via a micromanipulator, has further refined these procedures.

Minimal access surgery to the nose and paranasal sinuses

Surgery of the nose, paranasal sinuses, and anterior skull base has been revolutionised by the application of computed tomography and the rigid nasal telescope.

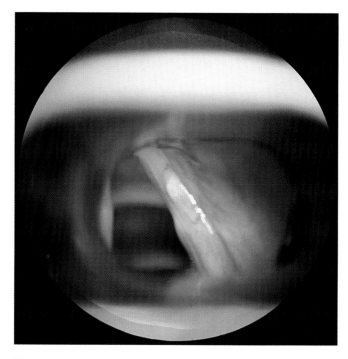

Figure 14.1 Laryngeal microsurgery. Endoscopic view of the right vocal fold, with a patch of leukoplakia visible on its upper surface

Computed tomography, particularly in the coronal plane, shows all the paranasal sinuses, especially the intricate and highly variable anatomy of the ethmoid labyrinth and disease within its air cells (figure 14.3). It also shows the important surgical relationship of the ethmoid bone to the floor of the anterior cranial fossa, the orbit and, in axial views, the orbital apex. This detail is not apparent on plain sinus radiographs.

The rigid nasal telescope is a lightweight, hand held instrument using a Hopkins rod optics system with fibreoptic light illumination, providing a clear, magnified view of any part of the nasal cavity. The telescopes most often used are 4 mm or 2·7 mm in diameter, with optical viewing angles of 0, 30 or 70°. The telescope is used to illuminate and view the operative site while the surgical instruments (angled forceps, suction, scissors, et cetera) are introduced into the nose.

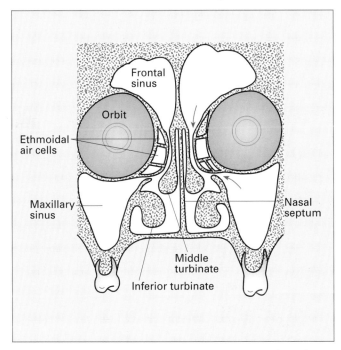

Figure 14.2 Nasal and sinus anatomy. Note how the frontal and maxillary sinuses drain via narrow channels (arrowed) through the ethmoid area to open lateral to the middle turbinate

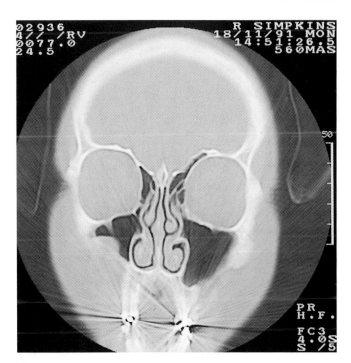

Figure 14.3 (b)

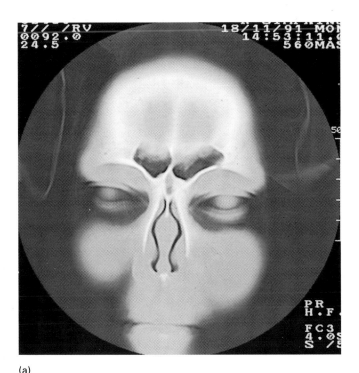

(a)

Figure 14.3 Serial coronal computed tomography sections through the nasal cavity, showing the normal frontal, maxillary and ethmoid sinuses. Note in (c) the close relationship between the ethmoid air cells, the orbit, and the floor of the anterior cranial fossa. Note also in (c) the narrow maxillary ostia, high on the medial wall of the sinus.

Use of the nasal telescope in diagnosis

Outpatient nasal endoscopy provides a better view of the nasal cavity than that obtained by conventional inspection with a headlight and nasal speculum. It is performed after spraying the nasal mucosa with a vasoconstrictor/local anaesthetic solution.

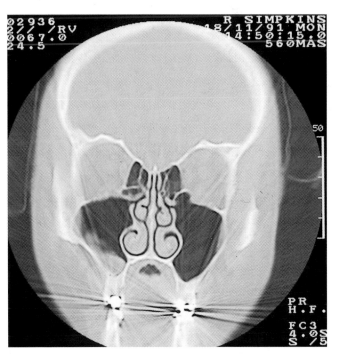

Figure 14.3 (c)

Blocked nose

For the patient presenting with a blocked nose, endoscopy can be used to identify the cause of obstruction: mucosal oedema, polyps, septal deformities, adenoid enlargement, or nasal tumours.

Recurrent or chronic sinusitis

In the assessment of recurrent or chronic sinusitis endoscopic inspection of the lateral nasal wall is very important. The middle meatus (a narrow cleft lateral to the middle turbinate) is the site of drainage of the frontal, maxillary and anterior ethmoid sinuses and obstruction here can predispose to infection. The obstruction may be caused by mucosal oedema or polyps and be aggravated by variations in normal

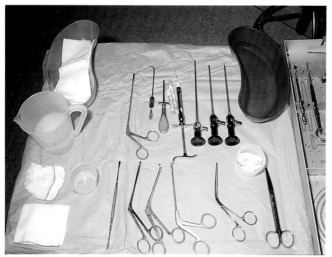

Figure 14.4 Telescopes and instruments for endoscopic sinus surgery

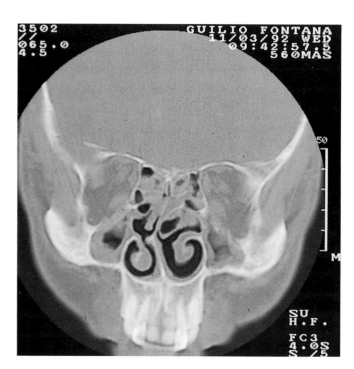

Figure 14.6 Coronal computed tomography of the sinuses in a patient suffering nasal obstruction and chronic sinusitis. Note the badly deviated nasal septum and opacified ethmoid cells

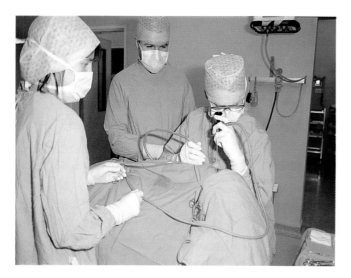

Figure 14.5 The nasal telescope in use

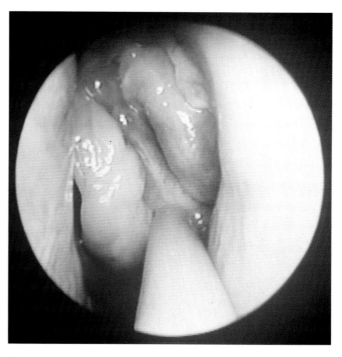

Figure 14.7 Nasal endoscopy: close up view of the right ethmoid area in the patient shown in Figure 14.6. The sucker is touching the middle turbinate. Grey polyps are visible to either side of the middle turbinate, obstructing sinus drainage

ethmoid anatomy that narrow the middle meatus (for example, pneumatisation of the middle turbinate). An accessory maxillary ostium, posterior to the main ostium, may interfere with normal mucociliary clearance from the antrum and predispose to infection. Messerklinger[1] described the role of these changes in the genesis of sinusitis and introduced the concept of minimally invasive "functional" sinus surgery, in which relatively minor intranasal surgery to the anterior ethmoid, sinus ostia and middle turbinate (the "ostiomeatal complex") could improve sinus mucociliary drainage. This could cure chronic maxillary or frontal sinusitis without direct intervention to the main sinus.

Facial pain

Interestingly, the ethmoid anatomical variations that predispose to sinusitis can also cause facial pain of "sinus" character in the absence of sepsis, perhaps by inducing pressure changes in the obstructed sinus or by mucosal contact between the highly pain sensitive middle turbinate and adjacent structures. Nasal endoscopy is thus worth while for the patient presenting with facial pain.

Conventional surgical approaches to the paranasal sinuses

Paranasal sinus surgery (apart from intranasal antrostomy) can not be performed transnasally without the nasal telescope, as headlight illumination does not allow adequate access or visualisation. An extranasal approach was therefore required (figure 14.8).

Maxillary sinus

The maxillary sinus (antrum) is traditionally explored using a Caldwell–Luc approach via a sublabial incision in the line of the oral mucosa over the canine fossa. A "window" is created in the antrum by removing bone. This approach may be associated with considerable morbidity, including numbness of the upper incisors (anterior superior alveolar nerve damage), paraesthesia or numbness of the upper lip (infraorbital nerve damage), or an oroantral fistula (if the incision fails to heal).

Ethmoid sinus complex

The ethmoid sinus complex may also be approached via a Caldwell–Luc incision but access is difficult and incomplete for the anterior ethmoid cells. Better access may be obtained by an external ethmoidectomy through a 3 cm incision at the medial orbital rim (Howarth or Patterson approach). This heals well but leaves a scar in the middle of the face. A similar incision, slightly higher on the superomedial orbital rim, provides good access to the frontal sinus by allowing removal of bone from the sinus floor. The entire ethmoid air cell system is accessible through the nasal cavity, but simple intranasal ethmoidectomy fell into disrepute due to poor visualisation of the posterior ethmoid anatomy, and a high risk of accidental surgical damage to the orbit or anterior cranial floor.

ostiomeatal complex in the lateral nasal wall. Techniques for this approach are well established, with generally good outcomes: even quite severe mucosal sinus disease often reverts to normal once proper drainage is established. As a consequence, the extranasal approaches are less commonly employed.

Anaesthesia

Endoscopic operations on the nose and paranasal sinuses may be performed using local anaesthesia and intravenous sedation and analgesia, or general anaesthesia. If general anaesthesia is preferred a topical preparation of cocaine or adrenaline should be applied to the nasal mucosa to induce vasoconstriction and lessen intraoperative bleeding.

Surgical access

Computed tomography provides a "map" of the anatomy, and the telescope allows accurate views of the site for surgery, so the ethmoid air cells may be safely removed intranasally using a variety of delicate bone instruments.[2] After excising part of the anterior ethmoid, the natural maxillary sinus ostium can be widened to drain or inspect the antrum. Surgery to the frontal sinus drainage area is also possible once the anterior ethmoid cells have been removed, but it is technically difficult, requiring angled viewing telescopes. The sphenoid sinus is less commonly involved in inflammatory disease; it can be opened by widening its natural ostium in the posterior nasal cavity or approached via the ethmoid.

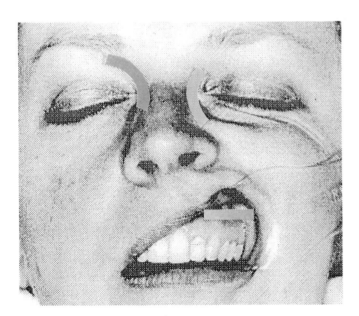

Figure 14.8 Extranasal approaches for sinus surgery. Red: frontal sinus exploration; green: external ethmoidectomy incision; orange: sublabial (Caldwell–Luc) incision for maxillary sinus exposure

"Minimally invasive" sinus surgery using the nasal telescope

The nasal telescope has changed the way in which sinus surgery is performed and Messerklinger's concept of "functional" surgery for sinusitis has directed surgery away from the major sinuses and focused on the

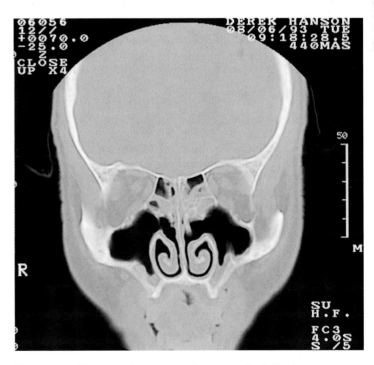

Figure 14.9 Postoperative computed tomography following endoscopic sinus surgery. The maxillary sinuses have been opened widely by removing the antronasal wall above the inferior turbinate (antrostomy), and are now healthy. However, the patient still suffers from purulent nasal discharge: the opacification of the ethmoid air cells indicates that this is due to unrecognised ethmoiditis

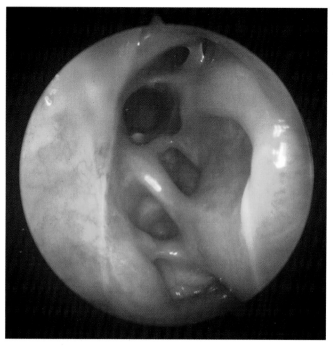

Figure 14.10 Postoperative endoscopy. This close up photo, taken with an angled endoscope, shows the roof of an ethmoidectomy cavity. A widely patent ostium leads upwards into the frontal sinus

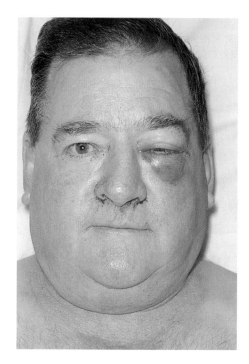

Figure 14.11 Orbital haemorrhage complicating endoscopic ethmoidectomy. The bruising became apparent 2 hours after surgery and settled spontaneously

Complications

- Orbital emphysema
- Cellulitis
- Avulsion of orbital structures
- Epiphora
- CSF rhinorrhoea
- Haemorrhage

Complications occur if anatomical barriers are transgressed. Violation of the lamina papyracea may result in orbital emphysema, cellulitis or avulsion of intraorbital structures. Damage to the lacrimal bone and nasolacrimal duct can cause epiphora. Cerebrospinal fluid (CSF) rhinorrhoea occurs if the roof of the ethmoid is damaged. Troublesome bleeding during surgery may necessitate packing the nose and abandoning the procedure for a later attempt. Serious reactionary haemorrhage can occur if the anterior ethmoidal artery is damaged; if the artery retracts into the orbit and continues to bleed urgent orbital decompression is required.

Extranasal approach

The extranasal approaches to the paranasal sinuses are not obsolete even though telescopes are in common use—they are still necessary for difficult cases with distorted intranasal anatomy due to disease or previous surgery, for complicated acute sinusitis (for example, orbital abscess complicating ethmoiditis), and for oncological resections. The Caldwell–Luc operation on the maxillary sinus is also part of the surgical approach to the pterygopalatine fossa, which lies posterior to the antrum. An external ethmoidectomy approach is commonly used for a transsphenoidal hypophysectomy,

in which pituitary tumours confined to the sella turcica can be excised under microscopic control without the need for a frontal craniotomy.

Use of the nasal telescope in other nasal procedures

Nasal/nasopharyngeal biopsy

Guided by the nasal telescope, outpatient biopsy of nasal and nasopharyngeal lesions is possible, preventing the need for inpatient admission for an examination under general anaesthesia.

Epistaxis

The telescope can be used to locate the bleeding point in some cases of severe posterior epistaxis, allowing local control with diathermy, and sometimes avoiding the need for nasal tamponade, which is uncomfortable for the patient.

CSF Rhinorrhoea

The management of CSF rhinorrhoea, spontaneous or posttraumatic, can be very difficult. The site of the leak may be in the cribriform plate, frontal, ethmoid or sphenoid sinuses and is not always visible on computed tomography. Traditionally, closure has been achieved via frontal craniotomy but if the leak is accessible to endoscopic surgery it might be closed intranasally. The leak is identified endoscopically and plugged with a free composite bone/mucosa graft taken from the inferior turbinate, secured in place by tissue glue and nasal packing.

Lacrimal surgery: endoscopic dacryocystorhinostomy

The lacrimal sac is another paranasal structure that is surgically accessible via the nose using the nasal telescope. Dacryocystorhinostomy (fashioning an opening between the lacrimal sac and nasal cavity) is undertaken to relieve epiphora or recurrent dacryocystitis due to lacrimal obstruction distal to the common canaliculus. It is usually performed using an external skin incision, but a recent report[3] indicates equivalent success rates using an endoscopic nasal approach. In an endoscopic dacryocystorhinostomy bone is removed from the lateral nasal wall just anterior to the middle turbinate to expose the lacrimal sac (figure 14.12). An opening is created and stented for several months with an indwelling tube.

Orbital decompression

Severe proptosis secondary to dysthyroid eye disease requires decompression of the orbit to prevent blindness. Removal of the ethmoid sinus and medial orbital floor, allowing inferomedial decompression, may be accomplished using an external ethmoidectomy approach, but this can be performed endoscopically by a transnasal approach, avoiding a facial scar. In endoscopic orbital decompression the ethmoid air cells are removed intranasally with the thin bony antronasal wall in the middle meatus, allowing access into the maxillary antrum. The orbital floor medial to the infraorbital nerve is removed with bone forceps, and the orbital periosteum incised to decompress its contents (figure 14.13).

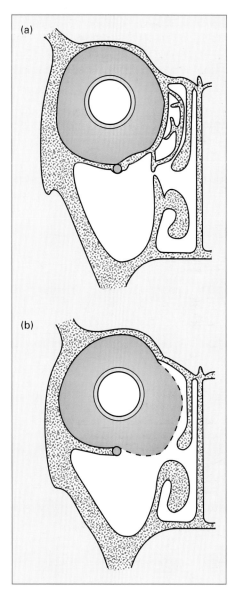

Figure 14.13 Endoscopic orbital decompression. (a) Before surgery; (b) postoperative view

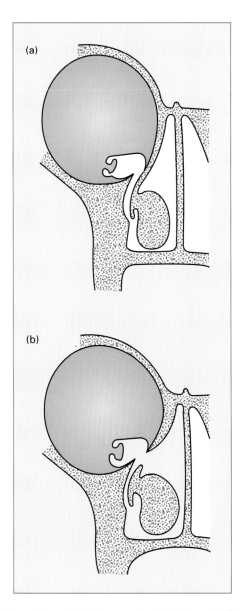

Figure 14.12 Endoscopic dacryocystorhinostomy. (a) The lacrimal sac normally drains tears via its duct into the nose, under the inferior turbinate; (b) at operation bone is removed medial to the sac, which is then opened directly into the nose

Future developments

The widespread use of the rigid nasal telescope has revolutionised the practice of surgical rhinology, allowing minimal access surgery to structures adjacent to the nasal cavity (paranasal sinuses, anterior cranial floor, lacrimal sac, orbit). Some of these "new" operations are widely practised, others are performed only in specialist centres. Laser technology is being applied to many of these procedures. Endoscopes are now available for the middle ear, but their impact on surgical otology remains to be seen. It is likely that, as new technologies become available, techniques become more reliable and new operations become incorporated into surgical training programmes, minimal access surgery of the ear, nose and throat will become more widely practised.

Acknowledgements

The author is grateful to Mr PR De for Figure 1, to Mr NS Jones for Figures 7 and 10, and to Mr NO Turner for advice in the preparation of the text.

1 Stammberger H, Wolf G. Headaches and sinus disease: the endoscopic approach. *Ann Otol Rhinol Laryngol* 1988;**97** (suppl 134):3–23.
2 Rice DH. Basic surgical techniques and variations of endoscopic sinus surgery. *Otolaryngol Clin North Am* 1989;**22**:713–26.
3 Metson R. Endoscopic surgery for lacrimal obstruction. *Otolaryngol Head Neck Surg* 1991;**104**:437–79.

In 1918 Professor Kenti Takagi[1] inspected the inside of a cadaveric knee with a cystoscope and is regarded as the first arthroscopist. The widespread clinical adoption of arthroscopy was slow but, with the development of smaller, more reliable fibreoptic scopes and improved instrumentation, arthroscopy of all the major joints has become an essential and established part of orthopaedic practice.

This chapter will consider the general principles of arthroscopy before reviewing its role in the assessment and treatment of pathology in individual joints. The reader is assumed to have the working knowledge of intra-articular and surface anatomy and pathology that is essential before embarking on any arthroscopic procedure.

Equipment

There is a bewildering array of arthroscopic equipment on the market, and the opinions of surgeons vary widely as to the amount and sophistication of equipment necessary. For most cases the set-up can be fairly simple.

A scope of 4·0 mm diameter with a 30° viewing angle (Figure 15.1) is used in the knee, ankle, shoulder and elbow; one 2·7 mm in diameter is used in the wrist. A scope with viewing angle of 70° is often used in the hip. The length of scope used varies, being longer for the hip and shorter for the wrist. The 30° viewing angle will usually give an adequate and complete view of the joint; however, 0°, 70°, and 120° scopes are available and are useful for visualising less accessible parts of the joint.

A camera is attached to the scope and the image displayed on a television monitor. This allows the operator to be in an upright and comfortable position throughout the procedure, and aids teaching. Integrated units, including a light source, camera, television monitor, video recorder, irrigation fluid pumps, and power tool links (if required) are commercially available and simplify operating room set up.

The number and design of arthroscopic instruments used is a matter of experience, necessity, availability and personal choice. Instruments are usually passed through a second portal some distance from the scope and the surgeon "triangulates" in order to view the instrument through the scope. As a rule, no instrument should be

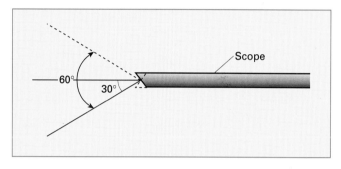

(a)

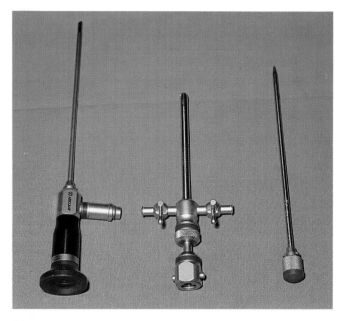

(b)

Figure 15.1 (a) A 30° viewing angle. By rotating the scope a 60° field of view can be obtained. Similarly, rotation of a 70° scope would produce a 140° field of view; (b) the trochar, cannula, and arthroscope

used within the joint unless its tip is clearly visible. The blind use of instruments is often the cause of surgical error.

A blunt hook is used to explore the joint, probing intra-articular structures, testing their integrity and, with

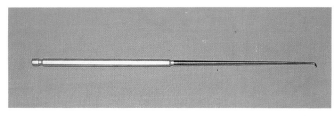

(a)

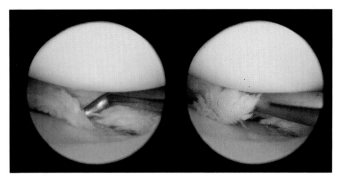

(b)

Figure 15.2 (a) A blunt hook; (b) the hook is used to probe a small tear in the meniscus

experience, feeling differences in tissue texture and consistency (Figure 15.2).

A variety of cutting instruments with different cutting angles and curves allows navigation around the contours of the bone permitting accurate placement, and precise cutting of tissues as required (Figure 15.3).

Grasping forceps are essential for retrieving surgical debris, loose bodies, and foreign bodies.

The introduction of powered instruments for shaving and resecting synovium, cartilage and bone has proven popular. Diathermy probes may be used for cutting and ablating tissue as well as securing haemostasis to good effect (Figure 15.4). Glycine solution must be used as irrigation if diathermy instruments are to be used. Carbon dioxide lasers have been developed for arthroscopic use.[2]

Such an array of equipment, combined with anaesthetic, nursing and surgical staff and the occasional need for radiographic monitoring, necessitates the use of a good sized, carefully laid out, operating area.

How to learn

Articular cartilage, once damaged or destroyed, has little or no potential for repair and the inexperienced arthroscopist can cause irreversible damage. A structured, sequential approach to training is therefore essential.

Observation in theatre, video recordings and well illustrated texts will give the novice an introduction to equipment, techniques, anatomy and intra-articular pathology.

Initial practice on model or cadaveric knees is useful for learning the siting of portals, insertion of scopes, basic techniques of positioning the scope within the joint, and finding the way around the joint. As experience increases models can be used to learn triangulation skills, and basic and advanced operative techniques without risking damage to a patient. A number of excellent courses for surgeons of all levels offer these facilities.

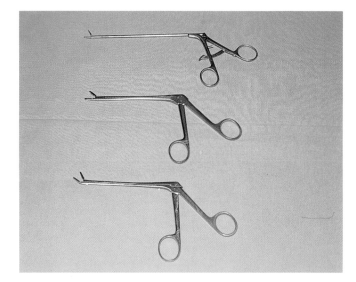

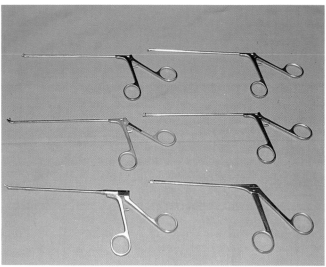

Figure 15.3 A range of instruments of different angles and curvatures is required for arthroscopic surgery

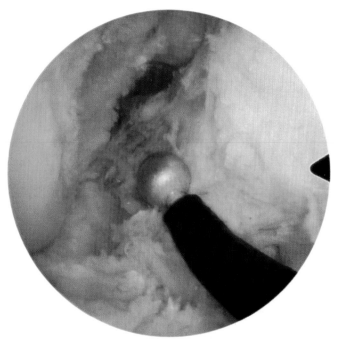

Figure 15.4 A diathermy probe securing haemostasis

Once a basic level of competence is achieved there is no substitute for well supervised teaching and experience in the operating room, preferably during a designated teaching arthroscopy list. Here the trainee has the time and opportunity to develop skills and increase the complexity of the procedures performed.

Anaesthesia

Many arthroscopies are performed under general anaesthesia; however, regional and local anaesthetic techniques are effective,[3] avoiding the complications of general anaesthesia—and the patient often enjoys watching their arthroscopy on the monitor. Injection of local anaesthesia into the wounds and the instillation of local anaesthesia or morphine into the joint at the end of the procedure decreases postoperative pain and aids rapid mobilisation and early discharge, particularly in day case patients.

Patient assessment

The diagnosis of any patient undergoing arthroscopy should be established before the procedure, if possible. A thorough and complete history and examination, complemented by appropriate imaging (plain radiographs, bone scan, arthrography, CT scan, CT arthrography, and MRI)[4] will establish the diagnosis in most cases. Arthroscopy is complementary to clinical assessment, not a substitute for it. The value of the information obtained must be weighed against the increased cost and morbidity of arthroscopy compared with other, less invasive, techniques.

Complications

One of the principal advantages of arthroscopy is its low morbidity. Complications do occur, but many are avoidable.[5]

- Anaesthesia related
- Diagnostic error
- Haemarthrosis
- Infection
- Compartment syndrome
- Intra-articular damage to:
  cartilage
  ligaments
  menisci
- Tourniquet causing:
  pain
  neuropraxia
  spirit burns
- Limb holders:
  ligament damage
  neuropraxia
- Traction injury:
  neurovascular
  muscular
  ligamentous
- Thromboembolic disease
- Vascular injury (direct)
- Instrument breakage
- Synovial fistula
- CO_2 extravasation

Tourniquets need not routinely be used. A solution of adrenaline (1:200 000) infiltrated around the proposed portals, and the use of a diathermy probe as required will keep the field clear of blood and reduce the incidence of haemarthrosis. If a tourniquet is used it should be sealed to avoid the ingress of alcohol based skin preparations, and the inflation pressure and time should be kept to a minimum and closely monitored to avoid neuropraxia and postoperative thigh pain.

Pressurised irrigation systems should be avoided in cases of possible capsular rupture as they carry a high risk of compartment syndrome subsequent to fluid escaping into the fascial compartments of the limb.

Close attention to operative sterility must be maintained with meticulous preparation, draping and theatre technique. Non-sterilisable equipment (such as the camera) must be excluded by sterile covers.

Careful wound closure with adhesive paper sutures will reduce wound leakage and infection and improve cosmesis. Portals must be accurately placed and carefully made to avoid the risk of inadvertent intra-articular damage caused by over zealous "stab incisions". Likewise, careful, controlled passage of instruments into and around the joint reduces the extent of articular cartilage scuffing. All instruments (manual, powered, diathermy, or laser) must be used only under direct vision, with the tip clearly in view, if accidental damage of intra or extra-articular structures is to be avoided.

Instruments and scopes must move freely in the joint. If they do not the reason for the obstruction should be sought and overcome by trying a different manoeuvre, a different instrument, or a different portal. Brute force has no place in arthroscopy and should not be used to push instruments or scopes into position as joint damage or instrument breakage will inevitably result. Should an instrument break, resulting in a loose fragment, the irrigation should be turned off and the fragment kept in view while thought is given to the best strategy for its removal, the appropriate instruments brought to hand, and a portal selected. The fragment should be removed carefully so that it is not displaced into a less accessible part of the joint. A magnetic probe (the "golden retriever") may be useful for removal of broken instruments.

Manipulation of the joint and traction should be carefully controlled, avoiding excessive force which could cause ligamentous injuries, traction injuries to nerves and vessels, or neuropraxias.

Only adequate training, practice and experience coupled with an ordered approach to each case will reduce diagnostic error to a minimum.

Audit

Controversies exist as to the value of arthroscopy in some areas (for example, the diagnostic accuracy of wrist arthroscopy compared with MRI or the benefit of arthroscopic versus open anterior cruciate reconstruction). All patients should be prospectively assessed and their outcome evaluated and carefully documented as part of an ongoing process of audit. Only by such a process will the true value and definitive indications of arthroscopy be established and unnecessary invasive procedures (with their associated morbidity) avoided.

Knee arthroscopy[6]

Examination under anaesthesia should always precede arthroscopy. The knee is inspected, evidence of any effusion sought and passive range of movements recorded. Integrity of the medial and lateral collateral ligaments and the posterior and anterior cruciate ligaments is assessed and tracking of the patella is observed.

The patient is placed supine and an abduction post positioned (Figure 15.5). A tourniquet is applied and sealed with adhesive exclusion drape, but should not be inflated. Local anaesthesia containing adrenaline (1:200 000) is infiltrated around the site of the proposed portals. The skin is prepared, including the toes and foot, and the patient is draped using a stockingette and crepe bandage to exclude the foot and lower leg.

The arthroscopic equipment is prepared and connected to the light source, monitor and irrigation. The surgeon should sit comfortably so that the leg may be manipulated into all the positions necessary for the procedure. The patient's hip is slightly abducted to allow the leg to overhang the edge of the table and the foot rests in the surgeon's lap. This permits control of flexion, extension and abduction during the procedure.

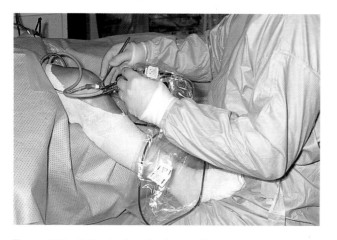

Figure 15.5 Patient set up for knee arthroscopy

The scope is introduced through the anterolateral portal (Figure 15.6), which is identified by pushing a thumbnail into the depression above Gerdy's tubercle and making a transverse incision 1 cm long just above, and as close as possible to the lateral edge of, the patellar tendon. The incision is deepened through fat, capsule and synovium, taking care not to incise articular cartilage, meniscus or the anterior cruciate ligament.

The cannula is inserted on the blunt trochar, initially directing it towards the centre of the notch but once it is in the joint directing it superiorly into the suprapatellar pouch. The trochar is removed and the presence and nature of any effusion or haemarthrosis noted and sampled if necessary. If blood or fluid is present the joint should be drained and thoroughly washed out before inserting the scope. A scope with a 30° viewing angle is introduced via the trochar and irrigation fluid run in to distend the joint. Once a clear view is obtained the examination can begin.

With the knee slightly flexed the suprapatellar pouch is inspected. As the scope is slowly withdrawn and rotated to look upwards the under surface of the

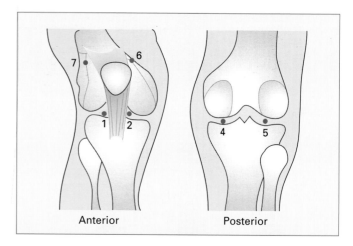

Figure 15.6 Portals used in knee arthroscopy (right knee): 1, anterolateral; 2, anteromedial; 3, central; 4, posteromedial; 5, posterolateral; 6, lateral suprapatellar; 7, medial suprapatellar

patella comes into view. Both facets are assessed, often aided by manipulation of the patella from side to side. Further withdrawing the scope, placing it obliquely across the knee and viewing superiorly, will reveal the patella and the trochlear groove. Flexion and extension of the joint will allow patellar tracking to be visualised. From this position the scope is swept over the anterior aspect of the lateral femoral condyle into the lateral gutter. After careful inspection the scope is swept across the front of the knee to the medial gutter.

From the medial gutter the medial femoral condyle is followed inferiorly towards the medial compartment. Valgus stress on the knee will allow inspection of the medial meniscus, tibial plateau, and femoral condyle. The view to the back of the knee is facilitated by positioning the knee in slight flexion only.

The scope is rotated to view the anterior horn of the medial meniscus and anterior joint capsule. A second portal is sited by passing a needle through the skin close to the patellar tendon just above the meniscus. By planning this portal under direct vision accuracy is assured. The needle is removed and a number 11 blade used to create the portal, again under direct vision to minimise the risk of intra-articular damage. A blunt hook may now be introduced to act as a probe, and the integrity of the structures in the medial compartment assessed (Figure 15.7).

The medial femoral condyle is followed laterally into the notch to inspect the anterior cruciate ligament (Figure 15.8), which is tested with the hook. If necessary the scope may be passed posteriorly to the medial or lateral side of the anterior cruciate ligament to view the posteromedial, medial and posterolateral compartments respectively. If further visualisation of the posterior compartments is desirable, posteromedial or posterolateral portals may be employed. The scope is withdrawn back into the notch and the lateral border followed inferiorly and laterally until the medial edge of the lateral compartment is seen. Keeping this in view the leg is brought into the "figure of four" position to apply a varus strain. The scope should now enter the lateral compartment with ease, allowing inspection and probing of the lateral meniscus,

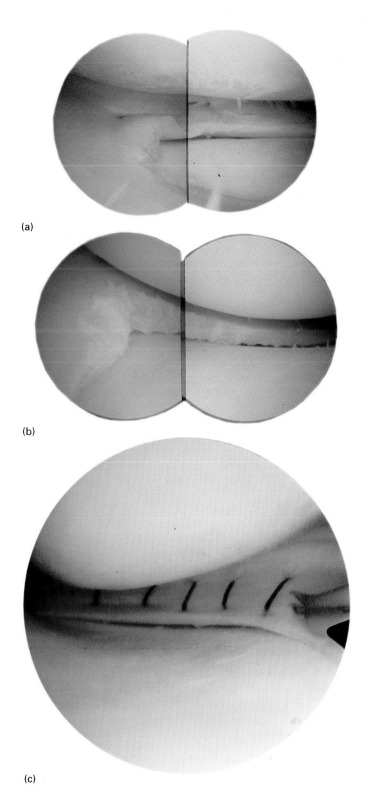

(a)

(b)

(c)

Figure 15.7 A small tear of the medial meniscus (a) has been arthroscopically resected using a punch (b). Peripheral tears that present early may be repaired using a meniscal suture (c)

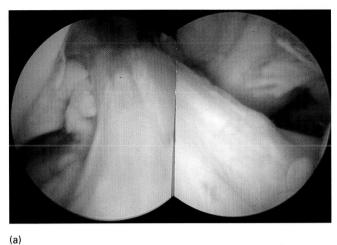

(a)

Lateral femoral condyle

Notch

Medial femoral condyle

Anterior cruciate ligament

(b)

Figure 15.8 View of the anterior cruciate ligament

found, procedure performed and the patient's functional parameters in conjunction with a physiotherapist.

Pathology and procedures

The details of the pathology that may be encountered, and the variety of procedures that may be performed, lie outside the scope of this book but are summarised in the box.

> ● Meniscal tear: partial menisectomy, repair (suture)
> ● Meniscal cysts: decompression
> ● Loose body: removal
> ● Osteoarthrosis: debridement, washout
> ● Synovitis: synovectomy, synovial biopsy
> ● Synovial tumour: synovial biopsy
> ● Synovial plicae: division
> ● Arthrofibrosis: adhesion division
> ● Osteochondritis: debridement, drilling, fixation, bone grafting
> ● Osteochondral fracture: reduction, fixation
> ● Intra-articular fracture: assessment of reduction
> ● Chondromalacia
> ● Maltracking patella: lateral release
> ● Anterior cruciate ligament rupture: reconstruction
> ● Posterior cruciate ligament rupture: reconstruction

popliteus tendon, and the lateral aspect of the tibiofemoral joint.

Once the arthroscopist is satisfied that the knee has been fully visualised and all amenable pathology identified and treated, the knee is irrigated and drained to remove any debris. Local anaesthetic is injected into the joint via the cannula and the cannula removed. The skin wounds are closed with adhesive paper sutures and a wool and crepe dressing applied.

An appropriate and structured programme of rehabilitation should be tailored to the pathology

Hip arthroscopy[7]

Arthroscopy of the hip is performed under general anaesthesia and preceded by examination under anaesthesia. Purpose made hip distractors are available but a standard fracture table will suffice. The patient is positioned and the theatre set up as in Figure 15.9. Traction is applied under image intensifier control to ensure that the hip joint will distract before commencing the operation. Traction is released while the surgeons scrub up and the patient is prepared and draped.

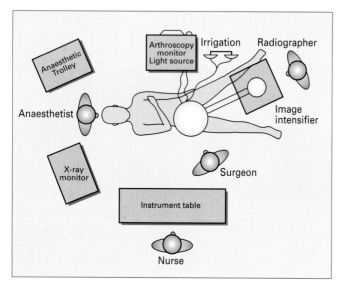

Figure 15.9 Layout of operating room for hip arthroscopy

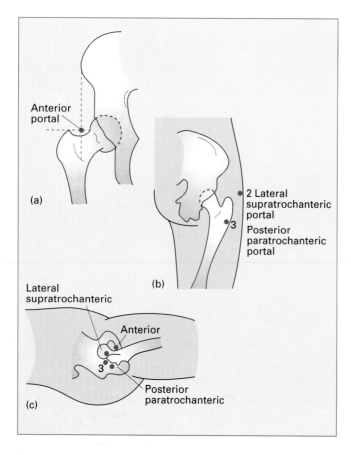

Figure 15.10 Portals used in hip arthroscopy (right hip). (a) Anterior view; (b) posterior view; (c) lateral view

Traction is reapplied and a hip aspiration needle is passed under the image intensifer control from the position of the lateral supratrochanteric portal (Figure 15.10). As the needle enters the joint the hip will distract as air is sucked into the joint. A guidewire is passed through the needle into the hip and the needle removed. A plastic scope cannula on a sharp cannulated trochar is passed over the guidewire under radiographic control until the trochar pierces the joint. The cannula is then pushed over the end of the trochar, further into the joint. The trochar is removed and a 70° scope introduced.

A second anterior portal is established in the same manner using a second plastic cannula. This is used for the passage of instruments and for setting up through and through irrigation if needed.

The sphericity of the femoral head, and the deep aspect of the hip joint, means instrument manipulation may be difficult and great care is needed to avoid joint damage or instrument breakage. Good views can be obtained (Figure 15.11) but the entire joint may not be visualised even if two or three portals are used.

Indications

- Diagnostic in undiagnosed pain
- Removal of loose bodies
- Removal of loose cement after hip replacement
- Synovial biopsy
- Synovectomy
- Osteoarthritis:
    Assessment
    Debridement and washout
- Osteochondritis:
    Resection
    Drilling
- Resection of labral tears
- Resection impinging ligamentum teres

Relative contraindications

- Avascular necrosis
- Congenital dislocation
- Ankylosis

Ankle arthroscopy[6]

Space in the ankle joint is limited and manipulation of instruments difficult. Adequate distraction of the joint eases this problem and can be achieved by the use of an external fixator with pins in the distal third of the tibia and the calcaneum and a distractor unit. The ankle is distended and saline injected via a needle placed in the joint at the position of the anterolateral portal (Figure 15.12).

The close proximity of neurovascular structures and tendons to the portals necessitates accurate placement of skin incisions and the deepening of the portals by spreading the soft tissues with dissecting scissors.

The scope cannula is inserted on a blunt trochar and the joint washed out. The scope is inserted and the anterior part of the talar dome, the distal tibia, and

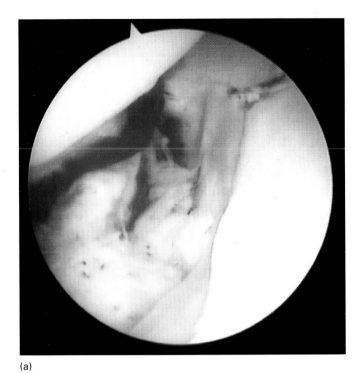

(a)

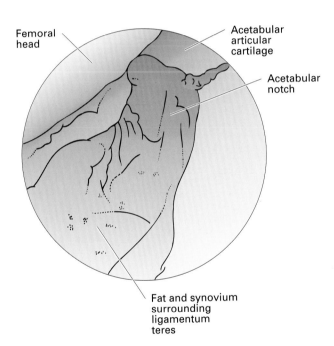

(b)

Figure 15.11 View of the acetabular notch

the medial and lateral malleoli can be inspected. If distraction is sufficient the scope can be passed between the talar dome and the tibia to view the ankle mortice. The curve of the talus will prevent a good view of the posterior joint: if this is required the posterior portals should be used.

The anteromedial portal is positioned by transilluminating the soft tissue anterior to the medial malleolus from within using the scope. This allows identification of the saphenous nerve and prevents damage during incision. This second portal can be used to pass a probe or other instrument or the scope may be inserted to gain a better view of the anterolateral side of the joint.

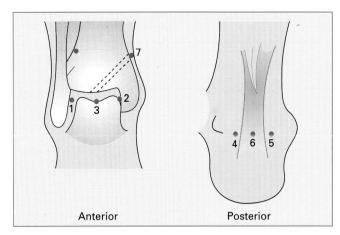

Figure 15.12 Portals used in ankle arthroscopy (right ankle): 1, anterolateral; 2, anteromedial; 3, anterocentral; 4, posteromedial; 5, posterolateral; 6, trans Achilles tendon; 7, transmedial malleolar (intraosseus)

Procedures

- Diagnosis
- Removal of loose body
- Osteoarthritis: debridement and washout
- Soft tissue impingement: resection
- Synovial biopsy
- Arthrodesis
- Osteochondral defects:
  Resection
  Drilling
- Assessment of intra-articular fracture
- Assisted stabilisation of instability

Shoulder arthroscopy[8]

After the obligatory examination under anaesthesia the patient is placed in the lateral position and traction applied (Figure 15.13). The operating room set up is similar to that for hip arthroscopy with the surgeon standing at the patient's back, but no image intensifier is needed.

The patient's skin is prepared and draped. A needle is inserted at the site of the posterior portal, 2 cm inferior to and 2 cm medial to the posterior angle of the acromium. It is directed towards a finger placed on the coracoid process (Figure 15.14). As the needle enters the joint air is sucked in and the joint distracts.

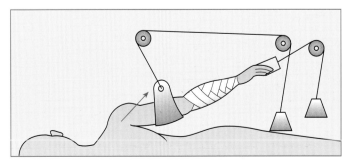

Figure 15.13 A method of applying traction to the shoulder. The resultant force is shown by an arrow

79

Irrigation fluid is injected to distend the joint. The arthroscope cannula is passed on the sharp trochar, taking care to avoid scuffing the articular cartilage. Irrigation fluid escapes as the joint is entered and the trochar is removed and replaced with the 30° scope.

A needle is passed from the site of the anterior portal, half way between the anterior edge of the acromium and the coracoid process, into the joint under direct arthroscopic vision. This allows through and through irrigation to be established. The anterior portal, for instrument introduction, must always be sited in the area lateral and superior to the coracoid process. A further superior portal may be sited in the angle between the clavicle and acromium, piercing trapezius.

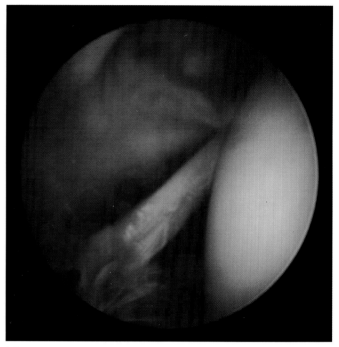
(a)

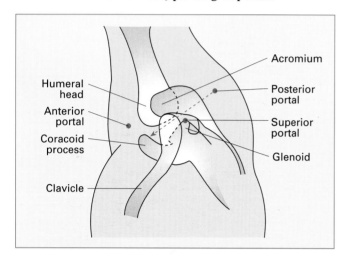

Figure 15.14 Portals used in shoulder arthroscopy

The joint is washed out using suction attached to a large bore needle. Once clear vision is obtained the joint is assessed in an ordered fashion.

Superiorly, the long head of biceps is identified. Above this the rotator cuff can be examined (Figure 15.15). The scope is slowly passed inferiorly to assess the anterior capsule, labrum, and glenoid. It is passed into the inferior recess and may then be withdrawn slightly and passed superiorly along the posterior labrum to view the posterior glenoid rim and posterior portion of the humeral head, including the bare area.

The arthroscope should also be used to examine the subacromial bursa. The same posterior skin incision may be used, passing the cannula on the blunt trochar more superiorly under the acromium until the scope rests on the coracoacromial ligament. The under surface of the acromium and the superior surface of the rotator cuff can be assessed.

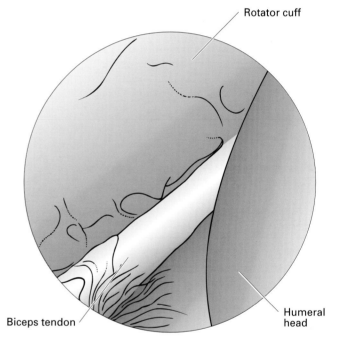
(b)

Figure 15.15 Arthroscopic view of the shoulder. There is a partial thickness undersurface tear of the rotator cuff

Pathology encountered

- Biceps tendon:
  Impingement
  Rupture
- Rotator cuff:
  Impingement
  Degeneration
  Tear
- Labrum tear
- Loose bodies
- Hill Sachs lesion
- Instability
- Subacromial impingement
- Osteoarthritis
- Synovitis
- Septic arthritis

Procedures

- Decompression of rotator cuff impingement
- Repair of rotator cuff tears
- Repair of labrum tears
- Removal of loose bodies
- Stabilisation of instability
- Decompression of subacromial impingement
- Debridement and washout of osteoarthritis
- Biopsy and synovectomy
- Washout of septic arthritis

Wrist arthroscopy[9]

Using a short 2·0 mm diameter scope good views of the radiocarpal and intercarpal joints can be obtained. Many portals have been described on the dorsum of the wrist and several may be used during one examination if the scope and instruments are to have access to both joints.

Wrist arthroscopy is a useful adjunct to radiographic investigations in selected patients with wrist pain and instability. It permits assessment of the intercarpal ligaments, articular cartilage and the triangular fibrocartilage complex (Figure 15.16). Techniques have been developed to resect or repair tears of this complex debride osteoarthritic joints and perform synovectomy. The arthroscope may also be used to assist in the reduction of intra-articular fractures and the repair of intercarpal ligament tears.

Elbow arthroscopy[6]

The close proximity of neurovascular structures, and the constrained nature of the joint, make access to the elbow difficult and the siting of portals must be precise. Several portals are required to permit evaluation of both anterior and posterior aspects of the joint.

Elbow arthroscopy is useful for the removal of loose bodies, debridement of osteoarthritis (arthroscopic O.K. procedure), assessment and treatment of osteochondritis, partial synovectomy, and synovial biopsy.

Other techniques

Endoscopic carpal tunnel decompression[10] has become popular with some surgeons, but opinion differs as to its relative efficacy and safety compared with the open technique.

Percutaneous techniques have been developed for removing prolapsed intervertebral discs[11] and good results may be obtained in selected patients.

As finer and more flexible scopes are developed more inaccessible areas, such as the epidural space and facet joints, are starting to come into the arthroscopist's field of view.

Acknowledgements

The following are thanked for their teaching, support, and help with illustrations: Mr M J Bell, Mr D Bickerstaff, Mr N Kehoe and Mr I Stockley, consultant orthopaedic surgeons, Sheffield; Mr R Calvert, consultant orthopaedic surgeon, St George's Hospital, London.

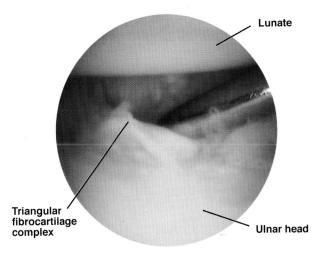

(a)

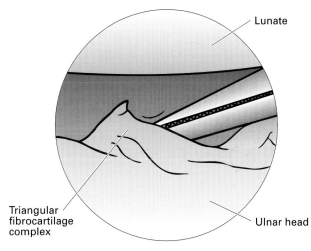

(b)

Figure 15.16 Arthroscopic view of the wrist. A tear of the triangular fibrocartilage complex is being probed

1 Takagi K. The classic: Arthroscope, Kenji Takagi, J Japan Orthop Assoc 1939, *Clin Orthop* 1982;**167**:6–8.
2 Duckworth MA, Marquez RA. Carbon dioxide laser arthroscopy. A new dimension in knee surgery. *AORN J* 1991;**54**:716–29.
3 Wallace DA, Carr AJ, Loach AB, Wilson MacDonald J. Daycase arthroscopy under local anaesthesia. *Ann R Coll Surg Engl* 1994;**76**:330–1.
4 Ruwe P, Wright J, Lawr Randall R, Lynch K, Jokl P, McCarthy S. Can MR imaging effectively replace diagnostic arthroscopy? *Radiology* 1992;**183**:335–9.
5 Bamford DJ, Paul AS, Noble J, Davies DR. Avoidable complications of arthroscopic surgery. *J R Coll Surg Edinb* 1993;**38**:92–5.
6 McGinty JB (ed.) *Operative arthroscopy.* New York: Raven Press, 1991.
7 Villar RN. *Hip arthroscopy.* Oxford: Butterworth-Heinemann, 1992.
8 Bunker TT, Wallace WA. *Shoulder arthroscopy.* London: Martin Dunitz, 1991.
9 Rettig ME, Amadio PC. Wrist arthroscopy: Indications and clinical applications. *J Hand Surg (Br)* 1994;**19B**:774–7.
10 Bande S, De Smet L, Fabry G. The results of carpal tunnel release: open versus endoscopic technique. *J Hand Surg (Br)* 1994;**19B**:14–17.
11 Kambin P. Arthroscopic microdiscectomy. *Arthroscopy* 1992;**8**:287–95.

Bibliography

Journals

Diagnostic and Therapeutic Endoscopy. Switzerland: Harwood Academic Publishers.
Endoscopic Surgery and Allied Technologies. Stuttgart: Georg Thieme Verlag.
Journal of Laparoendoscopic Surgery. New York: Mary Ann Liebert Inc.
Minimal Invasive Therapy. Oxford: Blackwell Scientific Publications.
Seminars in Laparoscopic Surgery. London: WB Saunders.
Surgical Endoscopy, Ultrasound and Interventional Techniques. New York: Springer International.
Surgical Laparoscopy and Endoscopy. New York: Raven Press.

Review articles

American Journal of Surgery 1991;**161**(3).
Baillière's Clinical Obstetrics and Gynaecology. Laparoscopic surgery. London: Baillière Tindall, 1989.
Macintyre IMC, Wilson RG. Laparoscopic cholecystectomy. *Br J Surg* 1993;**80**:552–9.
Reddick EJ. Laparoscopic abdominal surgery: an update. Overview of recent publications. *Endoscopy* 1994;**2**:493–501.
Steiner W, Aurbach G, Ambrosch P. Minimally invasive therapy in otorhinolaryngology and head and neck surgery. *Min Inv Ther* 1991;**1**:57–70.

Books

Arregui M, Sackier J, eds. *Minimal Access Coloproctology.* Oxford: Radcliffe Medical Press Ltd, 1995.
Arregui ME, Nagan RF. *Inguinal Hernia: Advances or Controversies.* Oxford: Radcliffe Medical Press, 1994.
Copcoat ʹMJ, Joyce AD. *Laparoscopy in Urology.* Oxford: Blackwell Scientific Publications, 1994.
Cuschieri A, Buess G, Perissat J. *Operative Manual of Endoscopic Surgery.* Berlin: Springer Verlag, 1992.
Gomella LG, Kozminski M, Winfield HN. *Laparoscopic Urologic Surgery.* New York: Raven Press, 1994.
Gotz F, Pier A, Schippers E, Schumpelick V, eds. *Colour Atlas of Laparoscopic Surgery.* Stuttgart: Georg Thieme Verlag, 1993.
Grochmal S, ed. *Minimal Access Gynaecology.* Oxford: Radcliffe Medical Press Ltd, 1995.
Hall FA, ed. *Minimal Access Surgery for Nurses and Technicians.* Oxford: Radcliffe Medical Press Ltd, 1994.
Hullea JF, Reich U, eds. *Textbook of Laparoscopy,* 2nd ed. Philadelphia: WB Saunders, 1994.
Krasna NJ. *Atlas of Thoracoscopic Surgery.* St Louis: Quality Medical Publishing Inc., 1994.
Rosin D, ed. *Minimal Access Medicine and Surgery. Principles and Techniques.* Oxford: Radcliffe Medical Press Ltd, 1994.
Rosin D, ed. *Minimal Access General Surgery.* Oxford: Radcliffe Medical Press Ltd, 1994.

Societies

Association of Endoscopic Surgeons of Great Britain and Ireland
Society for Minimally Invasive Therapy
Society of American Gastrointestinal Endoscopic Surgeons
European Association for Endoscopic Surgery

Index